Advances in Minimally Invasive Surgery

Edited by Andrea Sanna

Published in London, United Kingdom

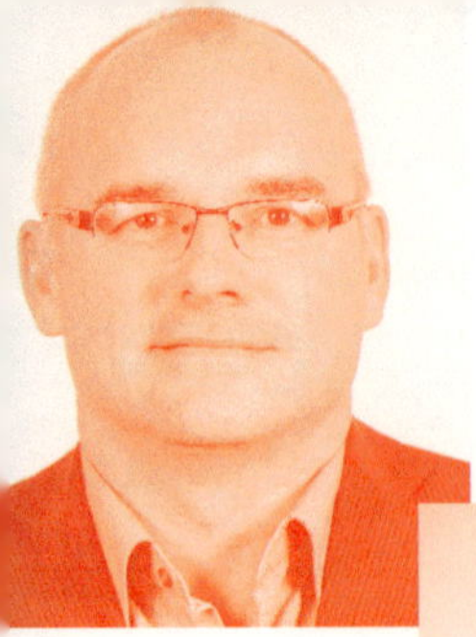
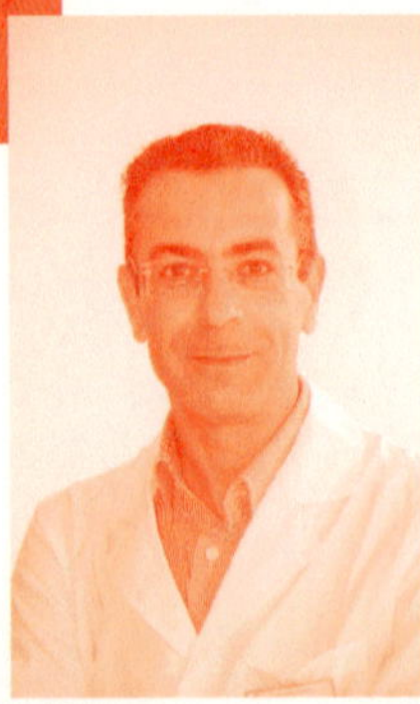
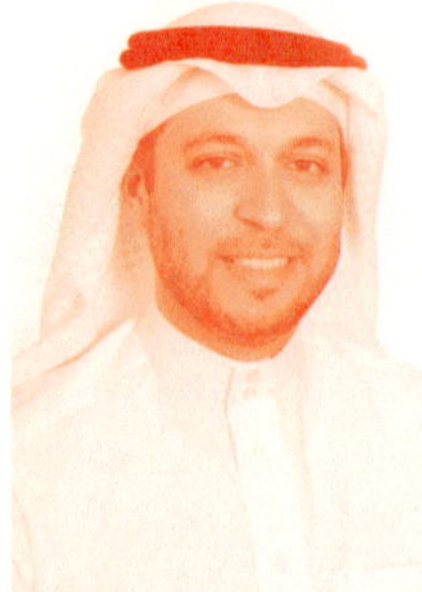
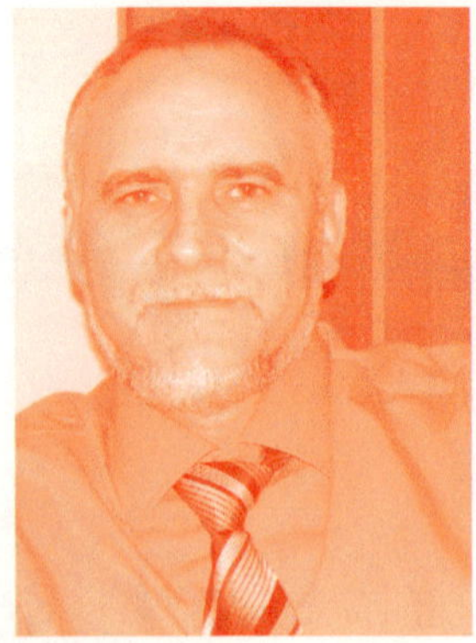
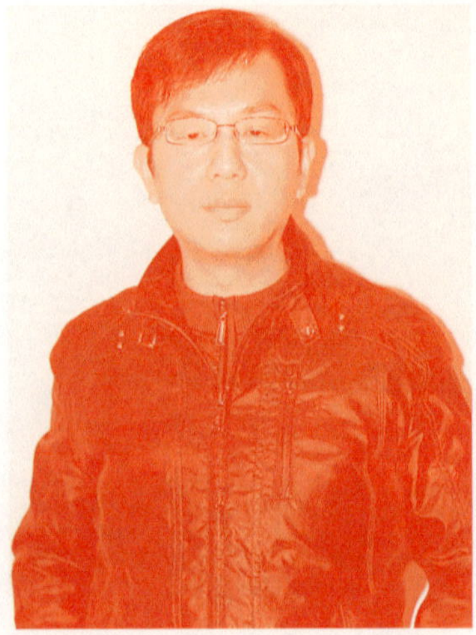
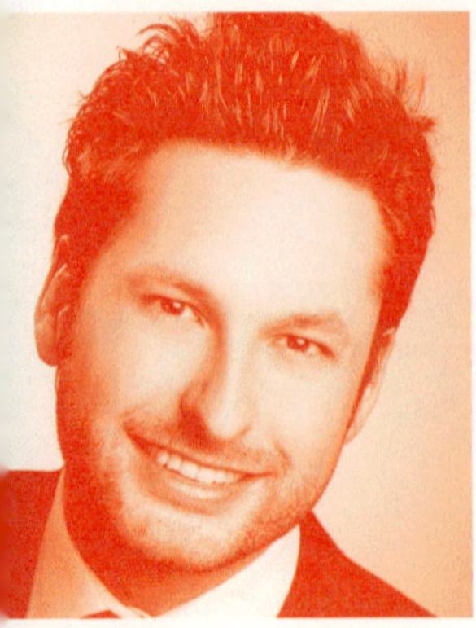
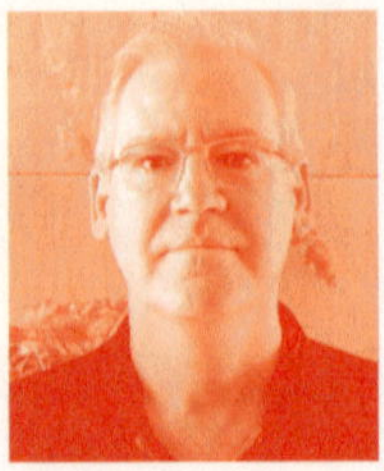

IntechOpen

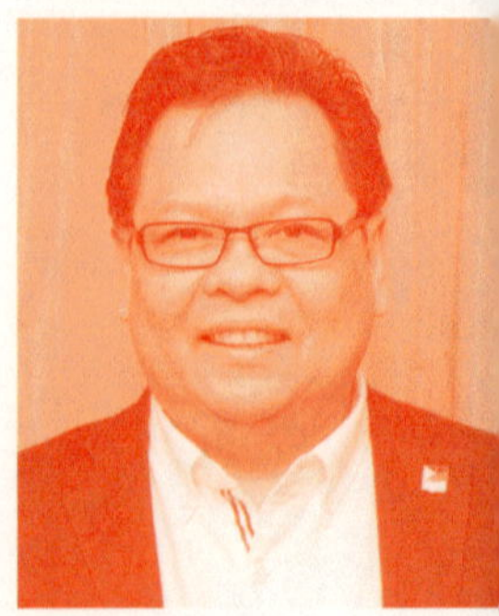
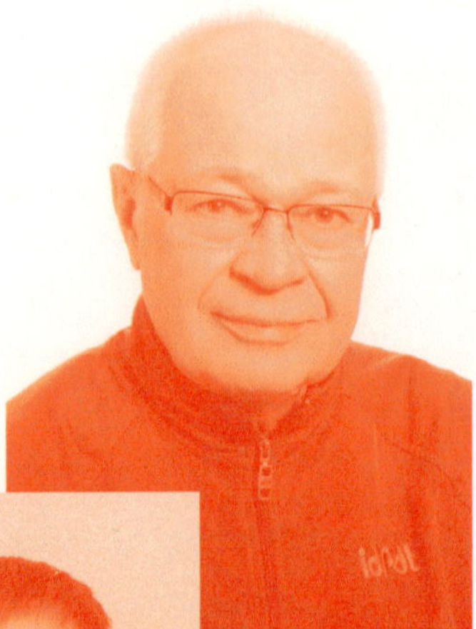
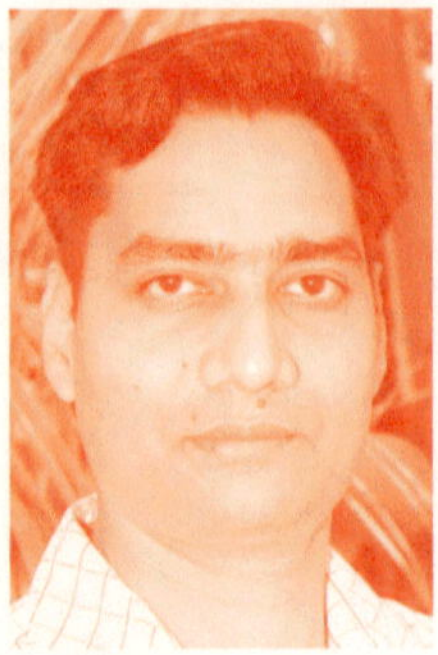
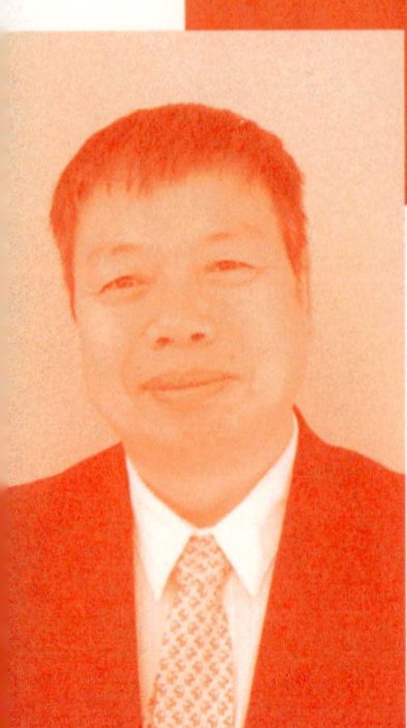
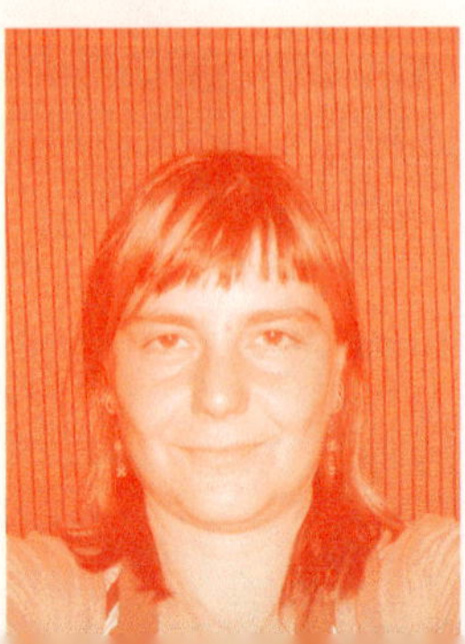
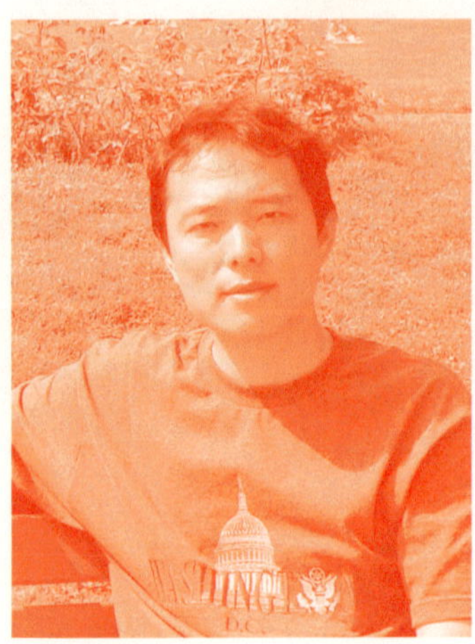

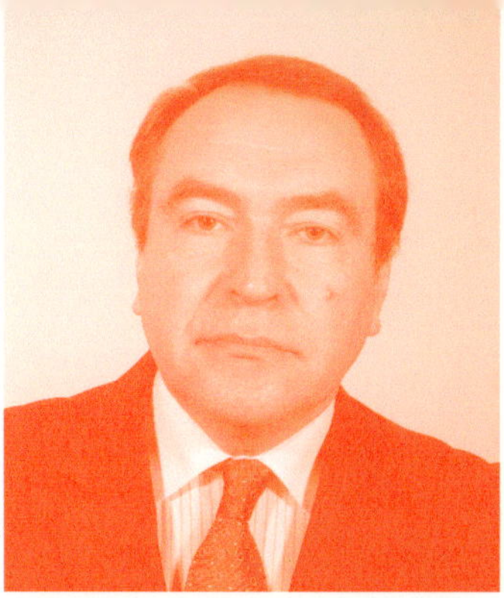
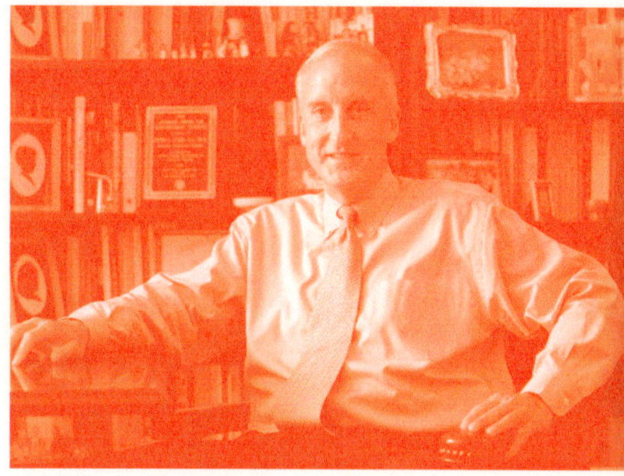
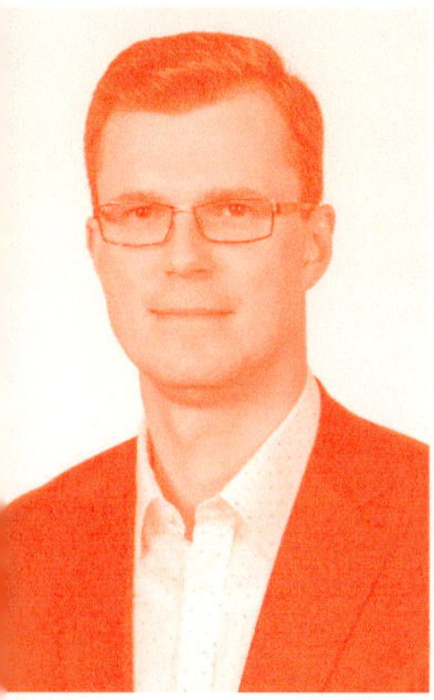
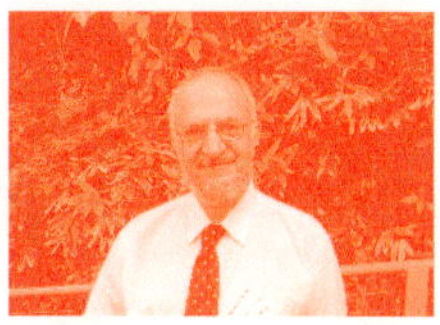
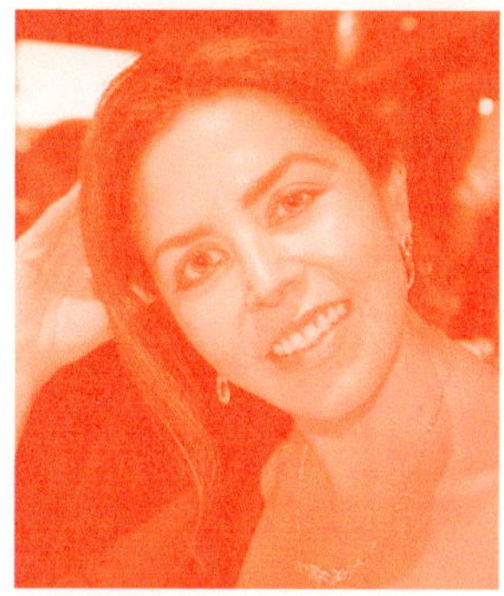

Supporting open minds since 2005

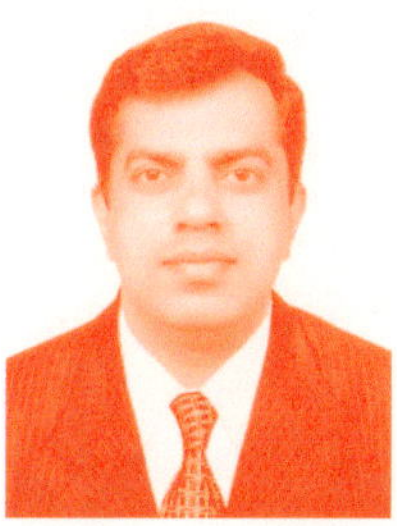
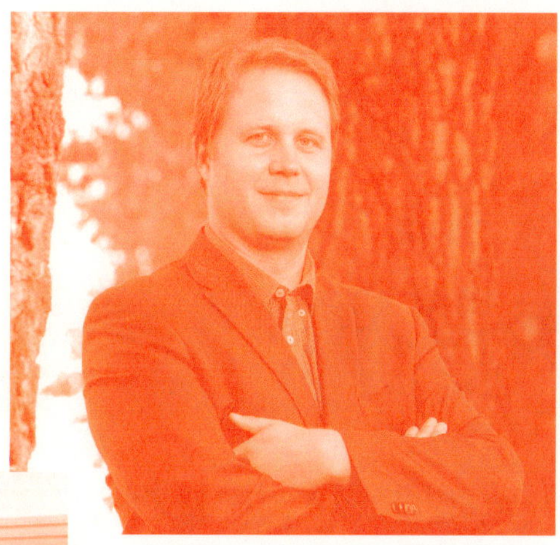
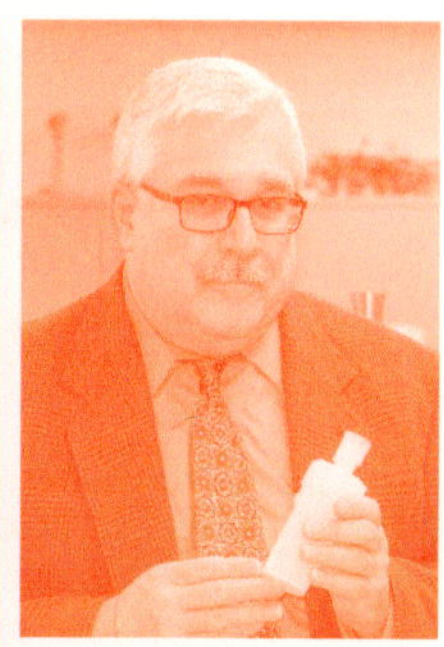
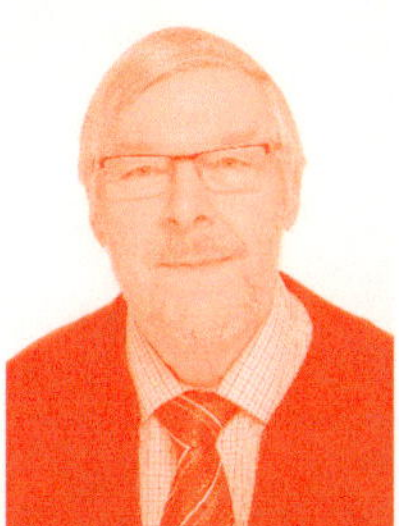
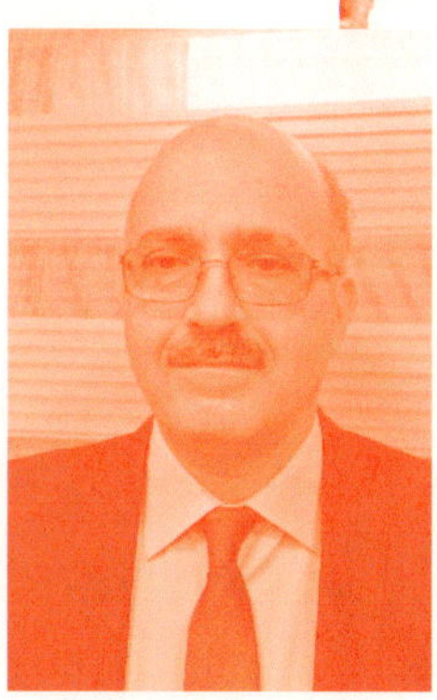
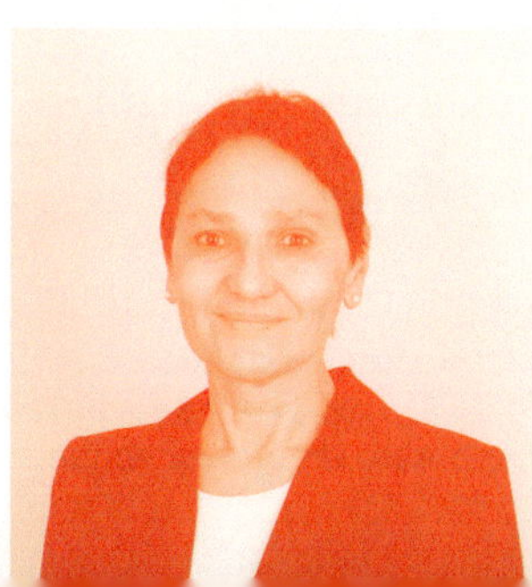
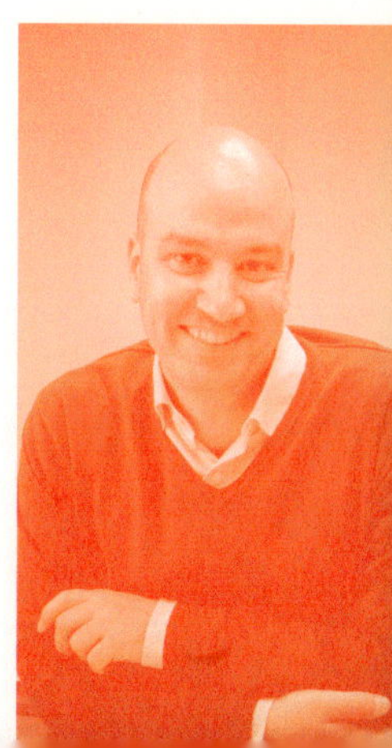

Advances in Minimally Invasive Surgery
http://dx.doi.org/10.5772/intechopen.92508
Edited by Andrea Sanna

Contributors
Andrea Papadia, Morena Antonilli, Vasileios Sevas, Maria Luisa Gasparri, Ammad Ahmad Farooqi, Ariel Revel, Shani Naor-Revel, Ruth Goldstone, Daniel Pereda, Elena Sandoval, Panagiotis Tsikouras, Christos Tsalkidis, Xanthoula Anthoulaki, Anna Chalkidou, Aggeliki Gerede, Stefanos Zervoudis, Anastasia Bothou, Spyridon Michalopoulos, Georgios Dragoutsos, Nikolaos Panagiotopoulos, Fotini Gaitatzi, Ioannis Tsirkas, Irini Babageorgaka, Theopi Nalbanti, Natalia Sachnova, Alexios Alexiou Constantinos Nikolettos, Sebidin Perente, Panagiotis Peitsidis, Nikolaos Nikolettos, Constantinos Nikolettos, Guntug Batihan, Kenan Can Ceylan, Juan Alberto Sánchez Margallo, Peter Gloor, David Durán Rey, José Castillo Rabazo, Carlos Plaza De Miguel, Manuel Ramón González Portillo, Isabel López Agudelo, Francisco M. Sánchez-Margallo, Andrea Sanna

First published in London, United Kingdom, 2022 by IntechOpen
IntechOpen is the global imprint of INTECHOPEN LIMITED, registered in England and Wales, registration number: 11086078, 5 Princes Gate Court, London, SW7 2QJ, United Kingdom
Printed in Croatia

British Library Cataloguing-in-Publication Data
A catalogue record for this book is available from the British Library

Additional hard and PDF copies can be obtained from orders@intechopen.com

Advances in Minimally Invasive Surgery
Edited by Andrea Sanna
p. cm.
Print ISBN 978-1-83962-572-5
Online ISBN 978-1-83962-573-2
eBook (PDF) ISBN 978-1-83962-574-9

For EU product safety concerns:
IN TECH d.o.o., Prolaz Marije Krucifikse Kozulić 3, 51000 Rijeka, Croatia, info@intechopen.com or visit our website at intechopen.com.

Meet the editor

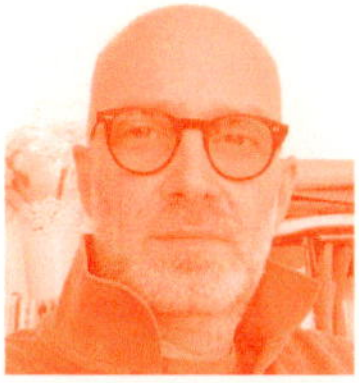

Andrea Sanna, MD, is a surgeon at Schiavonia General Hospital, Padua, Italy. He graduated in General Surgery from Ferrara University, Italy. His main clinical interests include minimally invasive techniques for the treatment of gastrointestinal cancer, abdominal wall reconstruction, and thyroid surgery. His areas of surgical specialty include laparoscopic colonic and gastric cancer; laparoscopic primary and incisional abdominal wall repair; extended-view, totally extraperitoneal primary and incisional abdominal wall hernia reconstruction; minimally invasive video-assisted thyroidectomy (MIVAT); and Desarda's groin hernia repair technique. Dr. Sanna has published several articles in peer-reviewed journals and authored several book chapters in general surgery. He is a member of several surgical associations including Associazione dei Chirurghi Ospedalieri Italiani (ACOI), European Hernia Society, and Società Italiana di Endocrinochriurgia (SIUEC).

Contents

Preface

Advances in Minimally Invasive Surgery is a collection of chapters concerning technology innovation in medical practice. It covers a wide range of applications of minimally invasive surgery in fields of medicine such as gynecology and cardiothoracic surgery. It also discusses advances in this surgical technique.

This book is written for healthcare professionals who wish to understand the principles and applications of new technology in minimally invasive surgery. Chapters are accessible to anyone, independent of prior technical knowledge. It is suitable as a textbook for undergraduate and postgraduate training in the clinical aspects of minimally invasive surgery, and as an introductory textbook for those pursuing a postgraduate career in surgical specialities.

I would like to thank the authors who shared their intellectual and practical expertise and experiences. I also want to thank the staff at IntechOpen, especially Ms. Maja Bozicevic and Ms. Iva Simcic, for their assistance, competence, and patience, without which publication of this book would not have been possible.

I hope that other experts will be encouraged to contribute to this work through their own experiences.

"Culture is the only good of humanity that divided between us all, instead of diminishing, will become greater." (Hans Georg Gadamer)

Andrea Sanna MD
UOC Chirurgia Generale-Departement of Surgery,
"Mother Teresa of Calcutta" Hospital,
Schiavonia, Padua, Italy

Section 1

Introduction

Chapter 1

Introductory Chapter: Advances in Minimally Invasive Surgery

Andrea Sanna

1. Introduction

If we want to beginning to describe the history of mini-invasiveness, we should write as a children's book "... once upon a time...". This is because the internal anatomy and pathology of the human body required direct visualization for centuries. The lightning source was the main limiting factor in applications of endoscopic or laparoscopic techniques. The Lichtleiter, described by Philipp Bozzini of Frankfurt in 1805, began the era of illumination. His cystoscope was the first example of inspection using a minimally invasive tool. Therapeutic applications of laparoscopy began in the 1930s by a gynecologist [1]. He initiated this process with the laparoscopic adhesiolysis using electrocautery in 1933. Subsequently, another gynecologist performed a tubal ligation using endoscopic electrocoagulation in 1936. Internists also appreciated the value of this technique using a peritoneoscope to increase their diagnostic accuracy. Laparoscopic cholecystectomy was the intervention that modified traditional surgery, giving impetus to the use of tiny incisions. Minimally invasive surgery has progressed in many surgical disciplines rapidly in the last 30 years [1]. It's know that there are evidence for the safety and efficacy of these approaches. The overall advantages as blood loss, hospital stay, pain control and surgical site infections (SSIs) has been know too in many of the MIS procedures compared with open surgery. Intuitively, patients' satisfaction has helped to drive the discipline of MIS. A rising number of MIS procedures have been exposed and integrated into surgical practice. The first MIS appendectomy was performed by a gynecologist (K. Seem). After this treatment, the attractiveness of this technique by the surgeons allowed to carry on the procedures forward by laparoscopic cholecystectomy in 1987 [1, 2]. Therefore, several surgical treatments became the new minimally invasive standard of surgical care. Consistency in benefits of MIS across procedures of different complexity and surgical subspecialty confers validity, as well as the adoption of MIS as an opportunity to improve quality. In the successful progress of MIS has been fundamentally the incessant achievement of technology equipment and the continuous development of instruments designed especially for this surgical approach.

2. Laparoscopic surgery

Laparoscopic surgery in humans has been developed since the first usage of peritoneoscopy, performed under direct vision to assess the peritoneal cavity, in the 1960s [1, 2]. The pioneers of video-assisted techniques were Semm K, with its laparoscopic appendectomy, and Muehe E, with its laparoscopic cholecystectomy. Those authors changed it from a diagnostic to a surgical procedure at the beginning of the 1980s, and it has since become a frequently applied technique for a wide field of indications. The procedure has become the standard practice for many surgical interventions performed in different medical fields [1, 2]. This technique has facilitated benefits such as a rapid recovery and shorter hospitalization, in addition to reduced postoperative pain. Despite the acceptance of laparoscopic surgery by a high number of surgeons in various types of abdominal surgery, many clinicians continued to express concerns that this technique would compromise survival by failing to achieve a proper oncologic outcome. After result, some trials demonstrated similar recurrence rates between laparoscopic and open surgery and suggested that laparoscopic surgery is an acceptable alternative approach to open surgery for the treatment of a high number of surgical conditions. It should be considered that minimally invasive surgery requires a longer learning curve than traditional surgery. This typically exhibits improvements in performance over time to ensure adequate outcomes and is an assist-dependent procedure [3–5]. Minimally invasive surgery has often been associated with both technical and technological advances attempting to overcome some limitations by combining open and laparoscopic techniques. For instance, hand-assisted technique was first introduced in the 1990s [1–5]. This technique, which provides excellent capabilities of exploration and safe specimen retraction, was useful because it allowed the use of laparoscopic instruments during colorectal surgery, splenectomy, and other procedures considered too complex for a laparoscopic approach. Unsurprisingly, the role of laparoscopy has increased in clinical practice. This move toward a minimally invasive approach can be seen with a decline in open surgical techniques in favor of percutaneous, endovascular, and minimally invasive interventions. Furthermore, laparoscopy has steadily and systematically become a dominant feature of today's general surgery trainees. Now that laparoscopy is progressively replacing open surgical approaches there may be some opposit problem. We think that for residents, it will become necessary to do learning curve in open surgery than in MIS.

3. Robotic

The da Vinci Standard surgical system was introduced early in the twentieth century. This robotic system was used in some field of surgery as urology, digestive surgery, and cardiothoracic surgery [5, 6]. The next-generation surgical system was introduced in the following years with field indications were enlarged as follows: general surgery, gynecology, and otolaryngology. In some countries, for laparoscopic surgery, the board certification system for physician was required. No board certification system exists in some countries for either society for robotic surgery, and this certification must be obtained from Intuitive Surgical Inc. Recommendations in guideline must start robotic surgery ideally with a single procedure, experience with several patients undergoing surgery, including observation and instructor-supervised surgery, and approval from a panel of experts for a single procedure (e.g., colorectal surgery or abdominal wall reconstructions). The robotic surgery usage increased dramatically from 2012 to 2018. It was found that the use of robotic surgery increased rapidly across numerous different procedures after hospitals begin performing robotic surgery. This trend was associated with a decrease in the use of laparoscopic minimally invasive procedures, which for most surgeons was already considered a safe and effective approach when clinically feasible [5, 6]. The advent of robotic surgery has certainly brought further advances in the field of mini-invasive surgery. However, it has been noted that many surgeons, due to the presence of the robotic platform in their hospital, have increased their use in various types of procedures. This trend has led to a decrease in the use of laparoscopy in some interventions, which for most surgeons was already considered a safe and effective approach when clinically feasible. It is believed that examining the costs of the method, the best use can be could be in fields where the limitation of laparoscopic surgery under difficult conditions such as a deep and narrow pelvis has overcome. Robotic surgery yields benefits such as dexterity of movement, a three-dimensional camera view, and reduced assistant-based physiological tremor.

4. Conclusion

The concept of minimally invasive surgery has been in our operating rooms for several years. New methods and new devices are used to minimize discomfort compared to open surgery. However, it should always be remembered that the complications of the new methods must be at least comparable to those envisaged by the standard open procedures.

Author details

Andrea Sanna
Department of General Surgery, Padova, Italy

*Address all correspondence to: and_sanna@yahoo.it

References

[1] Kaiser AM, Corman ML. History of laparoscopy. Surgical Oncology Clinics of North America. 2001;**10**:483-492

[2] Harrell AG, Heniford BT. Minimally invasive abdominal surgery: Lux et veritas past, present, and future. The American Journal of Surgery. 2005;**190**:239-243

[3] Khan N, Abboudi H, Khan MS, Dasgupta P, Ahmed K. Measuring the surgical 'learning curve': Methods, variables and competency. BJU International. 2014;**113**:504-508

[4] Rodríguez-Sanjuán JC, Gómez-Ruiz M, Trugeda-Carrera S, Manuel-Palazuelos C, López-Useros A, Gómez-Fleitas M. Laparoscopic and robot-assisted laparoscopic digestive surgery: Present and future directions. World Journal of Gastroenterology. 2016;**22**(6):1975-2004. DOI: 10.3748/wjg.v22.i6.1975

[5] Lacy AM, Delgado S, Castells A, Prins HA, Arroyo V, Ibarzabal A, et al. The long-term results of a randomized clinical trial of laparoscopy-assisted versus open surgery for colon cancer. Annals of Surgery. 2008;**248**:1-7

[6] Buchs NC, Pugin F, Volonté F, Hagen ME, Morel P. Impact of robotic general surgery course on participants' surgical practice. Surgical Endoscopy. 2013;**27**:1968-1972

Section 2

Minimally Invasive Surgery Approaches and Gynecology

Chapter 2

Minimally Invasive Surgery in Gynecology

Morena Antonilli, Vasileios Sevas, Maria Luisa Gasparri, Ammad Ahmad Farooqi and Andrea Papadia

Abstract

The first laparoscopic procedure was performed by 1901 by Georg Kelling in dogs while the first laparoscopic procedure in humans was performed by Hans Chrisitan Jacobaeus in 1910. Minimally invasive surgery offers multiple advantages over conventional laparotomy and is associated with reduced estimated blood loss, a lower incidence of complications and a shorter hospital stay and recovery. Over a century later, the vast majority of surgical procedures in gynecology are performed via minimal invasive technique. These include laparoscopy, minilaparoscopy, robotic surgery, laparoendoscopic single site surgery (LESS) and natural orifices transluminal endoscopic surgery. In this chapter we review these surgical techniques, analyze the main differences among these techniques and comment on their advantages and disadvantages.

Keywords: Gynecology, Minimally invasive surgery, Laparoscopy, Robotic Surgery, Ergonomics, artificial intelligence

1. Introduction

Minimally invasive surgery (MIS) can be considered as the greatest surgical innovation over the past 30 years. The major change and innovation of this surgery was to entry inside the abdomen avoiding large incisions on the skin, without affecting the surgical result and safety. The first description of minimal invasive approach as part of an endoscopy is attributed to Phillip Bozzini in 1805, who has visualized the urethral mucosa with a simple tube and candle light. Pantaleoni in 1869 has performed the first gynecologic procedure identifying uterine polyps. In 1910, in Sweden Hans Christian Jacobaeus performed the first Laparoscopy using a Nitze cystoscope. Heinz Kal, a German physician was revolutionary when developing laparoscopy into a diagnostic and surgical procedure in the early 1930's. The use of gaseous distention with lithotomy Trendelenburg position was firstly conceived by a French gynecologist Raoul Albert Charles Palmer a pioneer of Gynecologic Laparoscopy. The use of "cold light" and fiberoptics were landmark innovations in the endoscopy development. These outriders of endoscopic surgery as well as several other scientists and physicians have led the crucial groundwork that has enabled modern gynecology surgeons to perform laparoscopy on a routine basis, with a variety of energy systems under increasingly ergonomic and efficient conditions. Over time variants of the conventional laparoscopic technique have been developed to improve post-operative pain, cosmetic results and minimized trauma to tissue. (Minilaparoscopy, LESS, NOTES). In addition, since the 1980s surgical robots have been developed to address the limitation of laparoscopy in term of two dimensional visualization, incomplete articulation of instruments and ergonomic limitations. The Da Vinci System developed by the Stanford Research Institute along with the Defense department comprises of three components: a surgeon's console, a patient-side cart with four robotic arms manipulated by the surgeon (one to control the camera and three to manipulate instruments), and a high-definition three-dimensional (3D) vision system. Articulating surgical instruments are mounted on the robotic arms, which are introduced into the body through cannula. The need for remote interventions led to create a project by the National Aeronautics and Space Administration (NASA) in 1970s and funded by the Defense Advanced Research Project Administration (DARPA), for astronauts and soldiers in battlefields. Surgical robotics were first used in 1985 in neurosurgery; applications soon followed in urology (1988), orthopedics (1992) and gynecology (1998). It is important to notice that both traditional laparoscopic and robotic surgery have been widely adopted prior to emergence of data supporting efficacy and safety, because of its clear advantages compared to conventional surgery.

The patient is placed in a supine lithotomy position. Trendelenburg position is typically used to properly visualize the pelvis by displacing the bowel loops in the superior abdominal quadrants. The correct positioning of the patient plays a crucial role in the laparoscopic technique in terms of neurologic injury, ergonomic surgeon positioning, and adequate access to the vagina, if necessary. The patient's legs are placed in booted stirrups and it is important to maintain moderate flexion at the knee and hip with minimal abduction or external rotation at the hip. The buttocks should be a few centimeters beyond the edge of the table to allow uterine manipulation. To prevent migration in Trendelenburg position there are different methods: egg-crate foam directly beneath the patient, a vacuum-beanbag mattress, or shoulder braces. A variety of uterine manipulators are available to displace the uterus to facilitate access to pelvic structures. To manipulate the vaginal cuff, for women without uterus, a sponge stick can be positioned in the vagina.

To date, numerous studies have shown the superiority of minimal invasive surgery over laparotomy in terms of perioperative complications, hospitalization and quicker return to normal activity. On the other hand it was initially evident that there was a longer operating time and steeper learning curve for the laparoscopic technique. Today a greater surgical experience of surgeons and innovation of instrumentation have enabled a time overlap of most surgical procedures. In addition, a careful assessment of the patients (comorbidities, BMI and body habitus, patient's surgical history, type of pathology: size, shape, and mobility) to allow an appropriate safe and efficient procedure is crucial.

2. Minimally invasive techniques and approaches

2.1 Diagnostic and operative laparoscopic surgery

The laparoscopic technique uses a laparoscope that is introduced into the abdomen by means of small incisions on the skin (into or near the umbilicus) and that projects the images on an external screen. The laparoscope consists of a camera and a light source. Thanks to the gas insufflation inside the abdominal cavity, the operating space is increased for better visualization of the operating field and instruments. To date we have a wide range of laparoscopic instruments that mimic the ones used in conventional laparotomy. Two or three additional accesses are required for most surgical procedures. In gynecological surgery, usually the ancillary trocars are placed 2 cm medial and cranial to the lateral iliac spines, lateral to the inferior hypogastric artery [1–5].

Laparoscopes range from 1.8 mm to 12 mm in diameter having a distal end available in different angles. The 0-degree telescope is most commonly used and provides a straightforward view. While in contrast, a 30-degree fore-oblique lens allows for visualization in a large frontal view. Light is introduced through the laparoscope with a fiber optic cable powered by a light source. The camera unit consists of camera head, cable and camera control. The image resolution is dependent on the number of pixels on the chip. Most laparoscopic cameras have 250,00 to 380,000 pixels. Newer developments include the use of voice-activated, wireless systems designed to provide central control over operating room devices using either a microphone or a movable touch-pad screen.

Laparoscopy, as well as other endoscopic techniques, is based on two concepts that make it quite different from the open approach. These are triangulation and the fulcrum effect. Triangulation is a fundamental principle for endoscopic surgery as it allows to perceive the position of the instruments in three-dimensional space by sensing the position of our upper joints and arms across our chest together with visualization of the instrument tips (**Figure 1**). In fact, it is quite challenging to assess the distance or depth of the tip of a long instrument held in one hand. However, when a second instrument is used, the human brain can process the operative field visualized in the monitor with an impressive accuracy. Fulcrum effect is called the phenomenon where a handle movement of an instrument towards one direction is followed by a tip movement in the exact opposite direction. The tissue acts as a fulcrum or pivotal point. The tip movements ability and the right force needed to perform it, depends on the distance of the middle sign of the length of the instrument from the pivotal point according to the rules of physics (rule of moments). In other words, if more than 50% of the instrument length is beyond the fulcrum point, the tip movements are forceless and with a greater spectrum of movements (**Figure 2**) compared with the position when most of the instrument length is below the contact with the tissue.

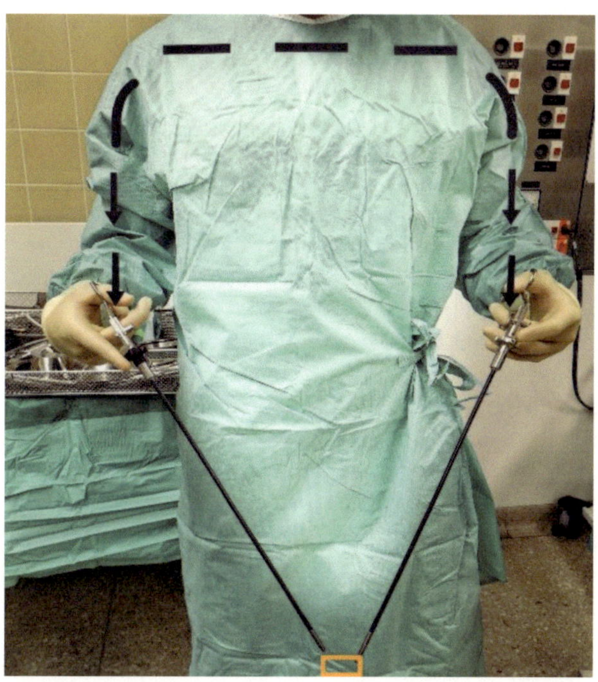

Figure 1.
Triangulation principle: the instrument will converge from different angles avoiding crossing and collision.

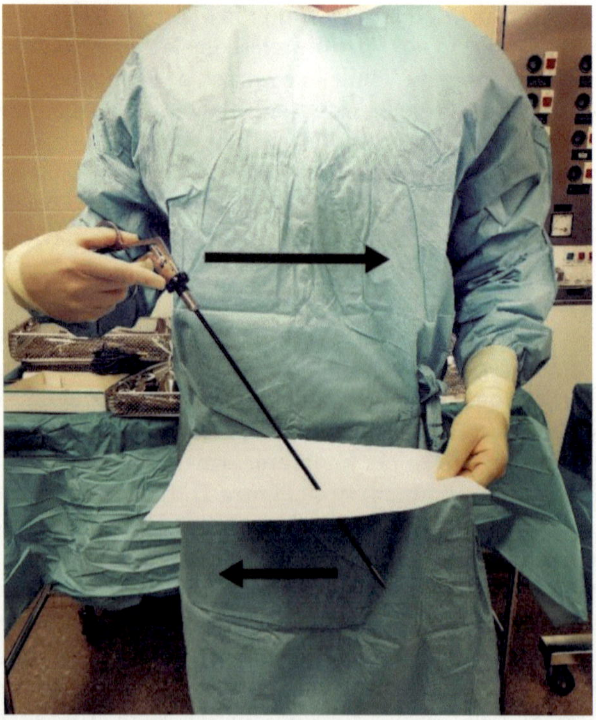

Figure 2.
Fulcrum effect: the abdominal wall, where the trocars are inserted, work as a fulcrum for the laparoscopic instruments. By moving the handle of the instrument to the left, through the fulcum effect, the tip of the same instrument will move to the right.

Gynecologic laparoscopic entry is commonly at or through the umbilicus. The traditional technique is to blindly pass a sharp Veress needle, at the umbilicus, insufflate, and then to pass a sharp trocar. Other closed technique entry, such as direct trocar entry, the radially expanding access system and open techniques are widely used. The method by which incisions are made to introduce the laparoscope may influence the likelihood of complications of the first step (injury to surrounding blood vessels or the bowel). However, a recent systematic Cochrane review comparing groups of patients undergoing laparoscopy with different entry technique, concludes that evidence is insufficient to show whether there were differences between groups in the rate of failed entry, vascular injury, or visceral injury, or in other major complications with the use of an open-entry technique in comparison to a closed-entry technique [6].

In general, complications of laparoscopy include nerve injury, vascular injuries, gastrointestinal injuries, trocar site hernia and urinary tract injury. Successful laparoscopy, just as in laparotomy, requires adequate visualization of the operative field and safe retraction of non-target tissues. An inability to displace bowel out of the pelvis, such as in morbidly obese women, and indistinct events such as acute intra-abdominal hemorrhage, may prompt a conversion to laparotomy. Poor candidates for laparoscopy are those with ventilatory problems, severe cardiorespiratory problems or elevated intracranial pressure as well as patients who cannot tolerate steep Trendelenburg or peritoneal insufflation.

2.2 Minilaparoscopy

Minilaparoscopy uses smaller abdominal incisions than contemporary laparoscopy and refers to the use of instruments and port sites of 5 mm or less. The 5 mm laparoscopes show high resolution and transport enough energy to properly illuminate the surgical field. These smaller port sites may be used for camera and/or accessory instruments (**Figure 3**). Although minilaparoscopy has been studied more extensively in general surgery and urology applications in gynecology have been described since 1991. A 3-mm incision was made for visualization with a plastic sheath. Two additional 3-mm incisions were used for accessory instruments to aid in adhesiolysis, biopsy of endometriosis, and laser myomectomy. The use of smaller instruments enhances the chance of decreased incisional pain, less need for post-operative opioid pain medication, shortened recovery time, minimization of tissue trauma, and provides a more favorable cosmetic outcome. One of the advantages that arise from minilaparoscopy in comparison with other forms of MIS is that it uses the same operating techniques, patient positioning, and instrument configuration as conventional laparoscopy. Few studies have shown contradictory results concerning operation time. No difference was proven in postoperative complications such as infection, conversion to laparotomy, reoperation, hospital readmission, estimated blood loss, and venous thrombosis although the literature in that field is still scarce [7]. Minilaparoscopy is an intriguing alternative to traditional laparoscopy and may gradually prove to be even superior.

2.3 Laparoendoscopic single site surgery

Laparoendoscopic single-site surgery (LESS), which is also called single-port surgery or single-incision laparoscopy is a procedure in which all instruments are inserted through a single skin incision, normally at the umbilicus (**Figure 4**). The first reported case of LESS was a gynecological procedure (tubal sterilization) performed by Wheeless in 1969. Approximately 20 years later, Pelosi et al. reported the first case of hysterectomy through LESS [8]. Currently, LESS is used in different surgical fields (general surgery, gynecology, urology). Compared with conventional laparoscopy, LESS shows substantial technical differences in procedure which, however, continue to be improved. These include: loss of triangulation and depth perception because the camera and working instruments are parallel to each other, limited extra-abdominal working space and decreased field of view due to suboptimal instrument or camera position. For this reason a specialized training is needed

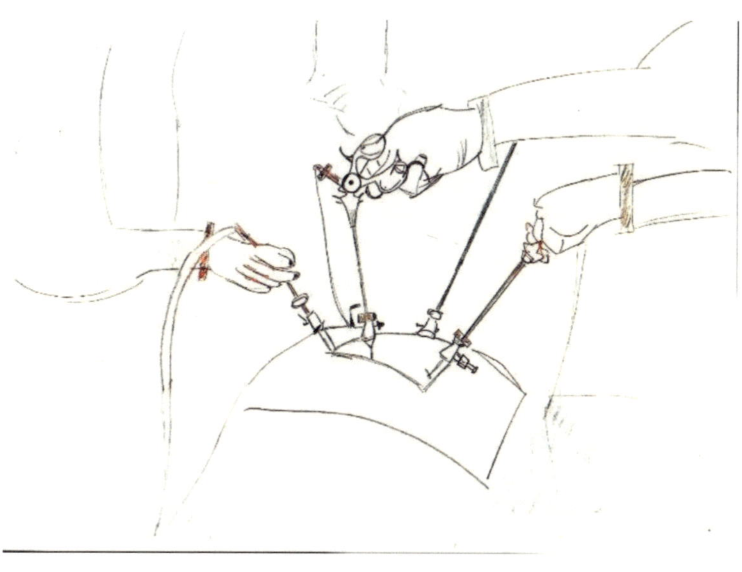

Figure 3.
Standard laparoscopy/Minilaparoscopy illustration: 3–4 entry sites are used on the abdomen for insertion of the instruments. The instruments will converge from different angles and will neither collide nor cross.

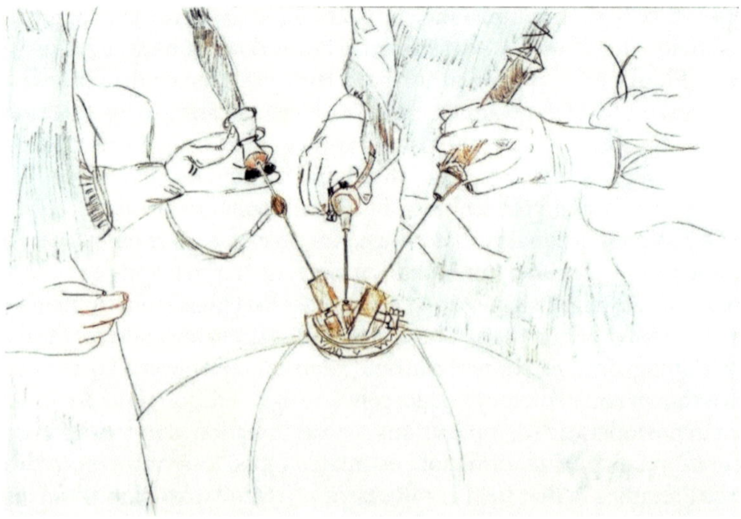

Figure 4.
Laparoendoscopic single-site surgery (LESS): a single port access is used and through this port, laparoscope and instruments are inserted. The instruments will cross at the umbilicus and will collide inside the abdomen.

to minimize these limits, but for surgeons experienced with standard laparoscopic techniques, adopting LESS seems to be feasible and safe. Essentially the advantage of this technique over the multiport laparoscopy would lie in the improvement of cosmesis, less pain, and decreased incisional morbidity. Recent data in gynecological surgery do not support the added of advantages of LESS over MLS. From an analysis of six randomized controlled trials (RCTs), conducted by Schmitt et al. in 2017 in patients undergoing LESS or MLS for adnexal pathology, there were no differences in length of hospital stay, blood loss, postoperative pain, and cosmetic outcomes [9]. In summary, the choice of LESS depends to a large extent on the skills and preferences of the surgeon after a thorough assessment of the morbidity of the patient and her pathology.

2.4 Natural orifice transluminal endoscopic surgery

Natural orifice transluminal endoscopic surgery (NOTES) has emerged as the newest concept of MIS (Minimally invasive Surgery) as an experimental alternative to conventional laparoscopy which provides an access to the peritoneum traversing a "natural" orifice (stomach, bladder, vagina, or rectum) with a multichannel endoscope [10]. When the procedure involves only transluminal access it is coined "pure" NOTES, compared with "hybrid" NOTES, which refers to a procedure performed through a natural body orifice with transabdominal assistance. The key technical elements in a NOTES procedure are access via a hollow viscus, performance of the desired maneuver once in the target cavity, and closure of the port upon exit. The choice of the entry site depends on the topography of the organ that must be subjected to surgery, considering a good visualization and proper manipulation of the instruments. For example, the trans-gastric pathway is appropriate for lower abdominal and pelvic procedures, while a trans-vaginal approach is preferable for upper abdomen organs. The conceptual bases that led to the development of NOTES have been the potential benefits of an incision of a viscus compared to the skin, the decrease in the risk of post-operative hernias and the obvious cosmetic result. On the other side, there are some limitations: many of the current instruments in use today are difficult to maneuver when the uterus is retroflexed.

Furthermore, a thorough closure of the viscerotomy is crucial to avoid bacterial contamination of the peritoneal cavity and abscess formation.

Of all the approaches, presently the transvaginal access to NOTES is the most common and seems to be the safest and most feasible for clinical application (**Figure 5**). Transvaginal NOTES (vNOTES) has been used for several operations other than cholecystectomy and appendectomy in humans. Potential complications of this approach include: dyspareunia, infertility, rectal and urinary injury. In 2012, Ahn et al. demonstrated firstly the feasibility and safety of vNOTES in gynecologic surgeries, which represented the key milestone in the evolution of NOTES [11]. The innovative and positive aspects of natural orifice surgery in gynecology include the lack of abdominal incisions, less operative pain, shorter hospital stay, improved visibility, and the possibility to skip lysis of adhesion to reach the pelvic cavity. However, for patients with severe adhesion and obliteration in the pouch of Douglas, vNOTES may be a contraindication due to higher risk of rectal injury. To date, two studies compared the surgical outcomes of vNOTES with conventional laparoscopic technique in gynecologic surgery. Both studies demonstrated that vNOTES could be safely performed for benign and large ovarian tumors and vNOTES might offer superior operative outcomes including blood loss, operating time and length of stay, compared to conventional laparoscopic technique [12, 13]. It seems obvious that sexual dysfunction may be an essential reservation of the females. Surprisingly, a study about transvaginal surgery has showed no problems of sexual intercourse and almost no cases of dyspareunia in a long-term follow-up [14]. The transvaginal peritoneal access for a gynecologist might not cause stress because of being familiar with the pelvic anatomy. Although transvaginal NOTES represents one of the most important innovations in surgery since the advent of laparoscopy, there are still technical limitations that must be overcome before the widespread use of this approach.

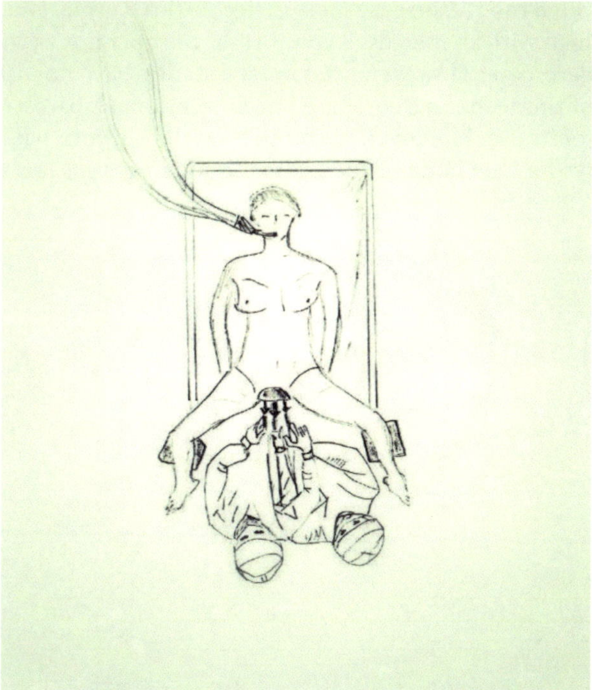

Figure 5.
Transvaginal natural orifice transluminal endoscopic surgery (vNOTES). An incision is made in the posterior vaginal fornix through which camera and instruments are inserted in the abdominal cavity.

2.5 Robotic surgery

Similar to laparoscopy, robotic surgery uses abdominal ports to create pneumoperitoneum to expand the operative field and to introduce the endoscopic instruments. The most known and currently the only commercially available system is the Da Vinci System (**Figure 6**). The patient is placed in the standard low dorsal lithotomy position with the legs supported in stirrups. One or two surgeon consoles are used to control robot arm movement. A separate robot column is positioned by the bedside and serves as the base for the four robotic arms. One of these arms controls the laparoscope while the other arms hold the robotic instruments. If port sites in addition to the basic four are needed, an assistant surgeon can operate by the patient bedside through one or two additional laparoscopic accessory ports. Port placement for robotic surgery is unique in that ports must be placed with a minimum interval distance of 8 cm. This makes sure that robot arms do not collide with each other and with any accessory port. Importantly, the depth of the inserted trocar in the abdomen is marked by a black ring around the cannula in order to adjust the right fulcrum during the operation. Robotic surgery presents significant technical advantages and some disadvantages compared with conventional laparoscopy. Advantages include 3D visualization of the operative field, mechanical improvement (instrument with seven degrees of freedom of movement), stabilization of instruments within the surgical field, and improved ergonomics. Disadvantages are mainly lack of tactile perception, increased cost, increased operating room time, large size of the devices and risk of mechanical failure. However, the robotic procedure is very useful and decisive in complex surgical procedures where extensive demolition is necessary with consequent restoration of the anatomy. In particular, the Endo Wrist technology is able to overlap with open techniques facilitating the execution of complex maneuvers even for the less experienced. Certainly, surgical simulation, tele-mentoring and telepresence surgery are potential novel benefits of robotic technology. Through robotic surgery most gynecological surgical interventions can be safely performed with an increased comfort for the operator as compared with conventional laparoscopy. However, randomized studies have not demonstrated the superiority of this technique compared to conventional laparoscopy and a clear indication of its use. Moreover, in comparison to conventional laparoscopy the learning curve for becoming proficient in robotic surgery is less steep and has

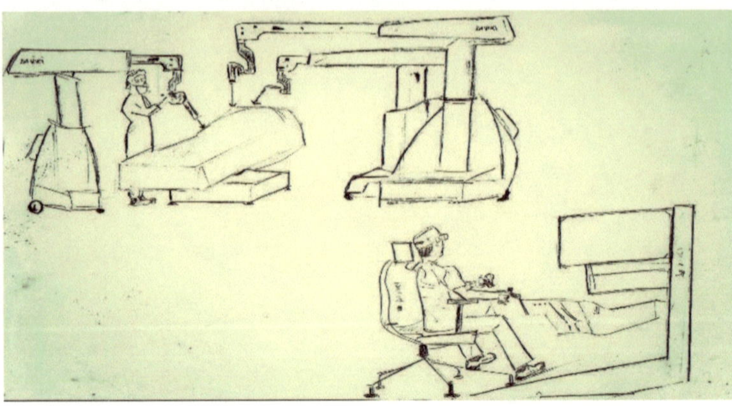

Figure 6.
Robotic surgery set up. It includes 3 components. A surgeon's console, a patient-side cart with four robotic arms manipulated by the surgeon (one to control the camera and three to manipulate instruments), and a high-definition three-dimensional (3D) vision system. Articulating surgical instruments are mounted on the robotic arms, which are introduced into the body through cannulas.

	Laparoscopy	Minilaparoscopy	LEES	Notes	Robotic Surgery
Advantages:	• Affordable cost • Proven efficacy in RCT's • Ubiquitus technology • Low post-operative pain • Good cosmetic result. Shortened recovery time	• Decreased incisional pain • Decrease in narcotic pain medication use • Minimization of trauma to tissue • More favorable cosmetic outcome	• Reduction in postoperative pain • Improved cosmetic outcome	• Lack of abdominal incisions • Less operative pain • No risk of post-operative hernias • No abdominal scars	• 3-D Visualization • Seven degrees of freedom • Tremor elimination • No fulcrum effect • Tele-surgery capability
Disadvantages:	• 2-D Visualization • Long learning curve • Limited degree of freedom • Reduced haptic feedback • Fulcrum effect • Amplified tremor	• Similar flaws to standard laparoscopic approach • More delicate and fragile laparoscope • Lower light quality and operative field visualization	• Slightly higher incidence of incisional hernia in comparison to multi-port laparoscopy • Restricted triangulation • Risk of external hand collision • Long learning curve	• Higher risk of rectal injury • Long learning curves. • Extended procedure times • Possible dyspareunia • Inability to deal with major complications	• High cost • Absence of touch sensation • Special training in specific centers. • Scarce proof of benefit on RCT's

Table 1.
Advantages and disadvantages of various types of MIS in Gynecology.

allowed a smooth transition to minimally invasive surgery for many gynecologists [15–20]. Last but not least, a newer Single Port Robot is currently available although not yet FDA approved for gynecologic procedures.

As it comes clear, nowadays there are various available minimally invasive techniques in the field of gynecology, each of them presenting specific advantages and disadvantages as shown below in **Table 1**.

3. Ergonomics in minimally invasive surgery

The term ergonomics derives from 2 Greek words: "Ergon" that means work and "nomos" that means law. In simple words it describes the science that prepares the worker to best fit his job by developing his working environment and necessary tools by offering the maximum favorable conditions [21]. Usually, when we talk about safety in the OR, anyone might be automatically thinking of safety concerning the patient and not the safety of medical and paramedical staff. Despite the proven safety and efficiency for patients, the development of laparoscopy came with exclusive ergonomic risks such as instrument length and handle design, inappropriate monitor position, and excessively high operating tables. Work-related musculoskeletal injuries and disorders are extremely common in the surgical staff with specific risk situations present in open, laparoscopic, vaginal, and robotic surgery. Needless to point out, that surgeon's safety has received scarce consideration, throughout the passage from laparotomy to MIS. Studies have shown that, despite significant impact of surgeon injury on productivity and career longevity, surgeons seldom and almost never report work-related injuries to the hospitals, building up a tendency of silent suffering. Although surgical ergonomics guidelines do exist, most surgical staff is not aware of guidelines, while targeted surgical ergonomics training is rare.

Work-related musculoskeletal disorders (WMSDs) as being the official term of this emerging phenomenon contribute immensely to reduced productiveness and job absenteeism. According to the guidelines, behaviors such as repetitions, application of more than 30% of strength, excess body segment positioning, prolonged static posture, use of vibration equipment and exposure to cold shall be averted. Given all that, it comes clear that WMSDs have the highest prevalence in the group of surgeons [22]. These sometimes inevitable movements could have important consequences to the admittedly long career life of a surgeon. Therefore, evidence based ergonomics training protocols should be available and become a compulsory part of residency programs to all teaching hospital around the world as it is well known, in the medical life but as well as in other scenarios bad habits hardly dissolve.

3.1 Ergonomics of conventional laparoscopy

The importance of ergonomics in the field of laparoscopy cannot be overemphasized. Studies have shown that ergonomics awareness and structured training can reduce chronic pain among surgeons as well as suturing time. The commonest sites of injury include the neck, back, shoulder, elbow, and wrist. This is no surprise as in comparison to conventional open surgery, in laparoscopy the surgeon presents prolonged static posture with no dynamic movements of the body resulting in decreased blood supply in the muscles and consequently elevated lactic acid and toxins in the blood circulation due to anaerobic metabolism. Moreover, redundant internal rotation of shoulder and deviation of elbow and wrist are more common in laparoscopy and have a huge impact in the mechanism of strain of the described regions. Risk factors for WMSDs include physician's traits such as younger age, shorter stature, female sex, smaller glove size, and higher volume, as well as higher patient BMI. On the other hand, protective factors include ergonomics awareness and training, excessive practice and higher surgeon age. Monitor position is a key component in laparoscopic surgery. Ergonomically, the ideal monitor position for laparoscopy is with the monitor image at or within 25 optimal degrees below the horizontal plane of the eye at a distance of approximately 60 cm. The same height, at which the video monitor used to be set for surgeons of different heights, has been demonstrated to be the underlying cause of neck pain and spondylosis in high-volume laparoscopic centers in the first decade after the onset of MIS in routine clinical practice [22–24].

3.2 Ergonomics of robotic surgery

Robotic surgery offers certain improvements in ergonomics such as greater degrees of freedom, motion scaling, tremor reduction, and 3-D immersive optics. Robotic equipment permits performance of fine tasks without the 'arcing' motions characteristic of conventional laparoscopy. Overall pain with robotics is decreased in comparison to open surgery and laparoscopy. Nevertheless, recent studies have questioned this demonstrated ergonomic advantage of robotics as McDonald et al. in 2017 concluded that robotic procedures were associated with more discomfort, stiffness and fatigue in a survey study of 350 surgeons [25]. Another study by Franasiak et al. has shown that approximately 45% of robotic surgeons experienced WMSDs while an impressive percentage of 26% showed to have experienced permanent damage. As resulted by the same study none of the observed surgeons reported injury to institutions while less than 17% of the total number had formerly received appropriate ergonomics training [26]. Given the rapidly emerging field of robotics in gynecologic surgery it comes clear that more solid evidence is needed in order to make safe comparisons between the ergonomic limitations of robotics versus laparoscopy [27].

4. Artificial intelligence and training the next generation of minimally invasive surgeons

Artificial intelligence (AI) and augmented reality have been steadily permeating the healthcare field and are expanding into gynecology. Although virtual artificial intelligence systems are still lacking in gynecology, gynecologic surgery has already integrated augmented reality (AR) technology into the operating room. For instance, cervical cancer models using AI have been used to foresee survival after surgery [28]. Over the past decade, gynecologic surgery has incorporated augmented reality in the form of computer-assisted or robotic platforms to close the native gap between open and minimally invasive surgical skills [29]. A.I applications range from simple prognostic tools to more complex models that incorporate clinical data, imaging, and histopathology to contribute into the optimal therapy decision. Various researchers argue that artificial intelligence is superior to traditional regression models in predicting outcomes. Another example of augmented reality in surgery is projecting preoperatively obtained radiologic images to the operating field during surgery to allow surgeons to understand the anatomical relationship between pathologic and healthy organs. Real time detection of the ureter during surgery is currently experimentally tested for eventual future use [30]. 3D printing is already reality in many centers and it permits advanced preoperative surgical planning and as a result minimizes potential injury. The most applicable example is by understanding the variation in uterine myomas where parameters such as size, location, and depth vary a lot and as a result 3D printing could guide the gynecologist to achieve an outstanding level of pre-op planning [31]. A recently published case report has had success in mapping endometriosis nodules with spatial organ involvement preoperatively with a 3DP model [32].

Virtual simulators have been recently utilized in training gynecologic surgeons for laparoscopic and robotic surgery. The simulator's efficacy has been assessed through published studies and has been shown to improve basic and advanced laparoscopic skills in all training levels. Novice residents improved their speed of execution, accuracy, and maintenance of horizontal view, while senior residents shortened their speed of execution. Virtual simulators could be incorporated into compulsory residency training as tools for practicing coordination and precision [33]. Hopefully we will reach to a point where as in aviation, it could become a requirement for novice trainees to practice and demonstrate adequate mastery of minimally invasive surgical skills before boarding on real surgery.

5. Conclusions

In conclusion, endoscopic approach remains the best choice in most of gynecological interventions. Despite the continuous groundbreaking advances in the medical technology concerning gynecologic procedures, the standard laparoscopic approach remains the universal king of the endoscopic gynecologic surgery. In everyday clinical practice, the final decision of the preferred technique depends on different variables: surgeon experience with the proposed technique, patient's characteristics and desire and finally costs. In particular, surgical costs can be divided into equipment costs and operating room time and surgical staff has to be more familiar with these costs as there is evidence that when surgeons are well informed and educated about operating room outlay, the cost of the procedure decreases. Moreover, the cost differential between robotic and laparoscopic hysterectomy decreases as surgeon and hospital volume increase [34]. For example, in selected cases such as hysterectomies for large uteri greater than 750 gr, robotic surgery has been shown to have cost-effective benefits compared to laparoscopic hysterectomy [35]. Minilaparoscopy, LESS and NOTES gave new perspectives to the minimal invasive conception, however despite of specific important flaws they are not frequently used into clinical practice up to date. Laparoscopic training as well as reduction of robotic-assisted technology costs by expanded use seem to be the constant for the future of minimal access surgery in the field of gynecology.

Conflict of interest

The authors declare no conflict of interest.

Author details

Morena Antonilli[1,2], Vasileios Sevas[1,2], Maria Luisa Gasparri[1,2], Ammad Ahmad Farooqi[3] and Andrea Papadia[1,2]*

1 Service of Gynecology and Obstetrics, Department of Gynecology and Obstetrics, Regional Hospital of Lugano EOC, Lugano, Switzerland

2 Faculty of Biomedical Sciences, University of Italian Switzerland, Lugano, Switzerland

3 Institute of Biomedical and Genetic Engineering (IBGE), Islamabad, Pakistan

*Address all correspondence to: andrea.papadia@eoc.ch

References

[1] Kaistha, Sumesh, et al. "Laparoscopic access: direct trocar insertion versus open technique." Journal of Laparoendoscopic & Advanced Surgical Techniques 29.4 (2019): 489-494. DOI: 10.1089/lap.2018.0408

[2] Boruta, David M. "Laparoendoscopic single-site surgery in gynecologic oncology: an update." Gynecologic oncology 141.3 (2016): 616-623. DOI: 10.1016/j.ygyno.2016.03.014

[3] Dorsey, J. H., and C. R. Tabb. "Mini-laparoscopy and fiber-optic lasers." Obstetrics and gynecology clinics of North America 18.3 (1991): 613-617.

[4] Ghezzi, Fabio, et al. "Minilaparoscopic versus conventional laparoscopic hysterectomy: results of a randomized trial." Journal of minimally invasive gynecology 18.4 (2011): 455-461 DOI: 10.1016/j.jmig.2011.03.019

[5] Acton, Jade N., et al. "Outcomes of total laparoscopic hysterectomy using a 5-mm versus 10-mm laparoscope: a randomized control trial." Journal of minimally invasive gynecology 23.1 (2016): 101-106. DOI: 10.1016/j.jmig.2015.09.001

[6] Ahmad, Gaity, et al. "Laparoscopic entry techniques." Cochrane database of systematic reviews 1 (2019).DOI: 10.1002/14651858.CD006583.pub5

[7] Layne, Alyssa Small, Lauren Pinkard, and Jessica Shepherd. "Current trends in minilaparoscopy." Current Opinion in Obstetrics and Gynecology 28.4 (2016): 255-260. DOI: 10.1097/GCO.000000 0000000290

[8] Pelosi, Marco A., and M. A. Pelosi 3rd. "Laparoscopic hysterectomy with bilateral salpingo-oophorectomy using a single umbilical puncture." New Jersey medicine: the journal of the Medical Society of New Jersey 88.10 (1991): 721-726.

[9] Schmitt, Andy, et al. "Single-port laparoscopy vs conventional laparoscopy in benign adnexal diseases: a systematic review and meta-analysis." Journal of minimally invasive gynecology 24.7 (2017): 1083-1095. DOI: 10.1016/j.jmig.2017.07.001

[10] Escobar, Pedro F., et al. "Laparo-endoscopic single-site and natural orifice surgery in gynecology." *Fertility and sterility* 94.7 (2010): 2497-2502. DOI: 10.1016/j.jmig.2017.07.001

[11] Ahn, Ki Hoon, et al. "Transvaginal single-port natural orifice transluminal endoscopic surgery for benign uterine adnexal pathologies." Journal of minimally invasive gynecology 19.5 (2012): 631-635 DOI: 10.1016/j.jmig.2012.04.001

[12] Wang, Chin-Jung, et al. "Natural orifice transluminal endoscopic surgery-assisted versus laparoscopic ovarian cystectomy (NAOC vs. LOC): a case-matched study." Surgical endoscopy 30.3 (2016): 1227-1234. DOI: 10.1007/s00464-015-4315-6

[13] Lee, Yi-Le, et al. "Transvaginal natural orifice transluminal endoscopic surgery for female-to-male transgender men." Journal of minimally invasive gynecology 26.1 (2019): 135-142. DOI: 10.1007/s00464-015-4315-6

[14] Mofid, Hamid, et al. "Is the transvaginal route appropriate for intra-abdominal NOTES procedures? Experience and follow-up of 222 cases." Surgical endoscopy 27.8 (2013): 2807-2812. DOI: 10.1007/s00464-013-2812-z

[15] Daiana, M., & Marescaux, J. (2015). Robotic Sugery. Br J Surg, *102*(2), e15-e28. DOI: 10.1007/s00464-013-2812-z

[16] Sinha, Rooma, et al. "Robotic surgery in gynecology." Journal of minimal access surgery 11.1 (2015): 50 DOI: 10.1007/s00464-013-2812-z

[17] Paraiso, Marie Fidela R. "Robotic-assisted laparoscopic surgery for hysterectomy and pelvic organ prolapse repair." Fertility and sterility 102.4 (2014): 933-938 DOI: 10.1016/j.fertnstert.2014.08.010

[18] Wright, Jason D., et al. "Robotically assisted vs laparoscopic hysterectomy among women with benign gynecologic disease." Jama 309.7 (2013): 689-698. DOI: 10.1001/jama.2013.186

[19] Orady, Mona, et al. "Comparison of robotic-assisted hysterectomy to other minimally invasive approaches." JSLS: Journal of the Society of Laparoendoscopic Surgeons 16.4 (2012): 542. DOI: 10.4293/108680812X13462882736899

[20] Sinha, Rooma, et al. "Robotic surgery in gynecology." *Journal of minimal access surgery* 11.1 (2015): 50. DOI: 10.4103/0972-9941.147690 DOI: 10.4103/0972-9941.147690

[21] Supe, Avinash N., Gaurav V. Kulkarni, and Pradnya A. Supe. "Ergonomics in laparoscopic surgery." Journal of minimal access surgery 6.2 (2010): 31.31. DOI: 10.4103/0972-9941.65161

[22] Catanzarite, Tatiana, et al. "Ergonomics in surgery: a review." Female pelvic medicine & reconstructive surgery 24.1 (2018): 1-12. DOI: 10.1097/SPV.0000000000000456

[23] Park, Adrian, et al. "Patients benefit while surgeons suffer: an impending epidemic." *Journal of the American College of Surgeons* 210.3 (2010): 306-313. DOI: 10.1097/SPV.0000000000000456

[24] Lee, Gyusung, et al. "Ergonomic risk associated with assisting in minimally invasive surgery." Surgical endoscopy 23.1 (2009): 182-188. DOI: 10.1007/s00464-008-0141-4

[25] McDonald, Megan E., et al. "Physician pain and discomfort during minimally invasive gynecologic cancer surgery." Gynecologic oncology 134.2 (2014): 243-247. DOI: 10.1016/j.ygyno.2014.05.019

[26] Franasiak, Jason, et al. "Feasibility and acceptance of a robotic surgery ergonomic training program." JSLS: Journal of the Society of Laparoendoscopic Surgeons 18.4 (2014). DOI: 10.4293/JSLS.2014.00166

[27] Stylopoulos, Nicholas, and David Rattner. "Robotics and ergonomics." Surgical Clinics 83.6 (2003): 1321-1337. DOI: 10.1016/S0039-6109(03)00161-0.

[28] Obrzut, Bogdan, et al. "Prediction of 5–year overall survival in cervical cancer patients treated with radical hysterectomy using computational intelligence methods." BMC cancer 17.1 (2017): 1-9. DOI: 10.1186/s12885-017-3806-3

[29] Sørensen, Stine Maya Dreier, et al. "Three-dimensional versus two-dimensional vision in laparoscopy: a systematic review." *Surgical endoscopy* 30.1 (2016): 11-23. DOI: 10.1186/s12885-017-3806-3

[30] Song, Enmin, et al. "A novel endoscope system for position detection and depth estimation of the ureter." Journal of medical systems 40.12 (2016): 1-11. DOI: 10.1007/s10916-016-0607-1

[31] Bourdel, Nicolas, et al. "Augmented reality in gynecologic surgery: evaluation of potential benefits for myomectomy in an experimental uterine model." Surgical endoscopy 31.1 (2017): 456-461. DOI: 10.1007/s00464-016-4932-8

[32] Ajao, Mobolaji O., et al. "Case report: three-dimensional printed model for deep infiltrating endometriosis." Journal of minimally invasive gynecology 24.7 (2017): 1239-1242. DOI: 10.1016/j.jmig.2017.06.006

[33] Paquette, Joalee, et al. "Virtual laparoscopy simulation: a promising

pedagogic tool in gynecology." JSLS: Journal of the Society of Laparoendoscopic Surgeons 21.3 (2017). DOI: 10.4293/JSLS.2017.00048

[34] Misal, Meenal, Ritchie Delara, and Megan N. Wasson. "Cost-effective minimally invasive gynecologic surgery: emphasizing surgical efficiency." Current Opinion in Obstetrics and Gynecology 32.4 (2020): 243-247. DOI: 10.1097/GCO.0000000000000636

[35] Moawad, Gaby N., et al. "Comparison of cost and operative outcomes of robotic hysterectomy compared to laparoscopic hysterectomy across different uterine weights." *Journal of robotic surgery* 11.4 (2017): 433-439. DOI: 10.1097/GCO.0000000000000636

Chapter 3

Minimally Invasive Surgical Treatment of Pelvic Pain in Teenagers and Young Women

Panagiotis Tsikouras, Christos Tsalikidis, Xanthoula Anthoulaki, Anna Chalkidou, Aggeliki Gerede, Stefanos Zervoudis, Anastasia Bothou, Spyridon Michalopoulos, Georgios Dragoutsos, Nikolaos Panagiotopoulos, Fotini Gaitatzi, Ionnis Tsirkas, Irini Babgeorgaka, Theopi Nalbanti, Natalia Sachnova, Alexios Alexiou, Constantinos Nikolettos, Sebaidin Perente, Panagiotis Peitsidis and Nikolaos Nikolettos

Abstract

Pelvic pain could be acute or chronic but rarely could be life threatening with various reasons such as pathological, physiological or functional. Clinical evaluation and management should be performed simultaneously, especially in emergencies that carry a high risk of mortality. Clinical evaluation and management should be performed simultaneously, especially in emergencies that carry a high risk of mortality. Although a detailed history, physical and gynecological examination, supplemented with imaging modalities can itself be diagnostic, the role of laparoscopy for diagnosis should not be overlooked. The common causes of pelvic pain with focus on a minimally invasive approach in this age group are as following: endometriosis, rupture of ovarian cyst, infection, ovarian torsion, pelvic vein syndrome, adhesions pain due to previous surgery and unsatisfactory treated infections.

Keywords: acute and chronic pelvic pain, gynecologic, non-gynecologic, endometriosis, cyst accident, torsion, ectopic pregnancy

1. Introduction

Pelvic pain is categorized as chronic or acute. Moreover should be mentioned that the incidence of pathology is different by age and it is essential to distinguish the causes that could be gynecological or non-gynecological. In adolescents appendicitis, cyst eruption or intussusception consist the most common causes of pelvic pain and on the other hand ectopic pregnancy, uterine fibroids, torsion of ovarian cyst, and pain are Mittelschmerz the most common causes of pelvic pain in women of reproductive age. Additionally, in postmenopausal woman diverticulitis, tumors and renal stones are the most frequent pathology.

There are multiple causes **of** pelvic pain with a broad spectrum of possible pathologies, physiological **processes** and functional syndromes that can cause pain. The pain is usually noncyclic. Chronic pain is defined as lasting for 3 to 6 months or more) [1]. The condition can be combined with abdominal pain. Contrary to the impression that chronic pelvic pain is usually related to gynecologic conditions, the majority of cases is related to gastrointestinal and urologic conditions [2]. Pelvic pain, in its severe form, can cause functional disability requiring an etiological or symptomatic treatment. Considering that the range of etiologies is diverse, both symptomatic and etiological management is often necessary. Among others, endometriosis, leiomyomas, adenomyosis, pelvic inflammatory disease and pelvic adhesions are included in the gynecologic conditions; interstitial cystitis, recurrent cystitis and recurrent urolithiasis are included in the urologic conditions; and irritable bowel syndrome, inflammatory bowel disease and celiac disease are included in the gastroenterologic disorders causing pelvic pain. Minimally invasive techniques could be proposed in both investigating and managing some of the above conditions. As an example, laparo-endoscopic single-site surgery technique could be considered in the management of endometriosis [1, 3]. Similarly, although routine laparoscopic adhesiolysis is not advised for pelvic adhesions, in selected cases, such as in one or two scars around an ovary, this specific adhesiolysis could be proved beneficial.

The surgical treatment of gynecological diseases in adolescence differs from that of adults. The way of coping with is affected by the high life expectancy and the necessity to maintain reproductive capacity [3, 4].

The sensitive psychology of adolescents should not be overlooked. Finding a mass inside the pelvis is an unpleasant experience at any age, but, in adolescence, is considered traumatic for both of the patient herself and her family [5, 6].

From the data of the international literature, which involve a large number of adolescent patients, it appears that:

- ovarian tumors are the most common tumors of the genital system at this age. Of these, 65% are benign, while 35% reveal signs of malignancy.

- Uterine body tumors are very rare in adolescence [3–7]. They are usually malignant and manifest with vaginal bleeding as the primary symptom.

- Tumors of external genitalia also have a low incidence, perhaps because the environmental factors that are causally related to their appearance have not yet been affected [8–12].

- In addition, vaginal and cervical tumors are very rare in adolescence.

A variety of gynecologic and non- gynecologic conditions such as approximately in 20% of cases endometriosis, pelvic inflammatory, adhesive disease, irritable bowel diverticulitis can lead to pelvic pain.

In this review is presented pelvic pain resulting from several gynecologic conditions and referred according to our experience [8–12].

2. Acute pelvic pain

Acute pelvic pain in this age group is characterized with the following symptoms: sharp, sudden pelvic pain, exacerbating pain with great intensity, short duration

(<24 hours) and usually occur in lower abdomen. In most cases, appeared also symptoms based on irritation of neural system like nausea, vomiting, sweating and tremor. Acute pelvic pain is the most often cause of visiting emergency department of gynecological clinic and it is a challenge for gynecologists for prompt diagnosis and treatment. The most often causes acute pelvic pain are as following [13–15]:

1. Causes that are not associated with pregnancy: pelvic inflammatory disease, degeneration of fibroids, ovarian torsion, cyst eruption, abscess.

2. Associated with pregnancy: ectopic pregnancy, miscarriage

3. Non- gynecological causes: appendicitis, diverticulitis, nephrolithiasis, inflammatory bowel disease, mesenteric lymphadenitis, typhlitis, gastroenteritis, bowel obstruction, cystitis, pyelonephritis, inguinal hernia, acute thromboembolic disease, coronary heart disease and abdominal aneurysm. Surgical treatment is most time with performance of laparoscopy or laparotomy, depending on the condition and the experience and training of the doctor [15–17].

3. Chronic pelvic pain (CPP)

Chronic pelvic pain is referred in pain has duration more than 6 months, occur lower abdomen and is associated to pain intensity great influence in life quality and sometimes requires multiple doctors visits and hospital admissions. The most common causes which could be functional, pathological, physiological are as following:

1. From gastrointestinal system

2. From urogenital system

3. From female reproductive system

4. From myoskeletal system

5. From neurological system

6. From psychological causes

Frequency is approximately 4–25%, however the minority of woman in this age group (33%) visit doctor.

Various studies have studied the incidence of chronic pelvic pain (CPP) in 5,000 women, aged 12 - -22 years, in the United States. In these studies, it was revealed that 15% suffer from CPP. Of these, only 10% visited a gynecologist, while 75% had no visits in any health care provider.

Despite the fact that such an increased number of women did not visit a doctor, CPP was the cause of 10% of gynecological visits, 10 - -40% of laparoscopic surgeries, and 10 - -16% of hysterectomies [18–23].

In the USA, every year are performed approximately 4000,000. If 10 - -16% of them done for CPP, then we could assume that 65000 to 104000 hysterectomies are performed due to CPP.

In addition, while the mortality of hysterectomies is about 0.1%, 65 - -104 of deaths can be attributed to surgeries for the treatment of CPP each year. About 35% had no visible abnormal CPP findings on laparoscopy. It is estimated that 58% of women limit their physical activity to at least one day a month, 10% seek for a doctor other than a gynecologist, while 1% seek for treatment with a psychiatrist [18–23].

The majority of the patients with chronic pelvic pain and negative laparoscopic findings (41%) were taken contraceptives, while 25% GnRH analogues for 3 months [18–23]. The American College of Obstetricians & Gynecologists recently argued that it is appropriate to prescribe empirical treatment with GnRH analogues for 3 months to women with CPP, without an exact diagnosis, who have not had any other anti-inflammatory drugs [18–23].

This approach is considered relatively safe and effective. If there is no response to this treatment, a laparoscopy or other surgical approach should be performed [18–23].

An empirical protocol is proposed by Winkel, which, after excluding other pathologies such as pelvic inflammatory disease or ovarian cysts, administers GnRH in proportion to an improvement effort. According to the results of various women, there is an improvement of 80% in patients with, or without, endometriosis, r17-22egardless of whether they have undergone laparoscopy or not [13–21].

4. Endometriosis

4.1 Definition and incidence

Endometriosis is characterized by the presence of endometrium outside the uterus, the proliferation and differentiation of tissue similar to the endometrium outside the cavity of the uterus. It is the one of most common cause of pelvic pain in women of reproductive age and the second most common gynecological condition after fibroids. Any peritoneal surface including tube ovary (where it may form endometriomas, peritoneal, bowel, bladder etc.

- If involving myometrium – adeno
- That it can be superficial, deeply infiltrating or form nodules. When penetration into fibrous tissue is revealed, the term external adenomyosis (adenomyosis, externa) characterizes this pathological condition due to its important similarity to adenomyosis (adenomyosis interna).

The term "“deep endometriosis” includes the morphological classification of endometriosis, which has a penetration depth greater than 5 mm [22–26].

The clear differentiation of deep endometriosis from other forms of the disease was observed by Donnez [24–28]. The nodular form of these lesions is due to the proliferation of smooth muscle fibers, their localization is retroperitoneal and may extend laterally to the anterior part of the rectum.

Although this entity is a common gynecological disease, responsible for 10 - -15% of infertility cases, little is known about the pathogenesis of the disease. For its etiology, several pathophysiological mechanisms have been proposed -, anatomical, immunological, endocrinological, environmental and finally genetic factors with genetic predisposition [24–28].

The genetic processes that regulate endometrial cell proliferation have not been fully elucidated. The etiology of endometriosis is unknown, but there is evidence to suggest that the genetic factor is associated with the development of endometriosis. The notion that endometriosis is a genetic disease was initially relied on poorly controlled studies in which a familial impact of the disease was found [24–28]. A familial tendency for endometriosis was first reported in 1957, but the first representative study of endometriosis genetics was conducted in Europe by Simpson et al.

in 1980 in Europe. It should be noted that relatives of second-degree patients had a 1.8% risk of endometriosis. Women with a family history of endometriosis tended to develop allergic reactions (eczema, asthma, allergic rhinitis). In addition, women with congenital endometriosis developed the disease at a younger age (mean age 22.1 years).

Finally, women with congenital endometriosis usually had the most severe form of the disease, the third and fourth stages of endometriosis, according to a revised American Fertility Society ranking. Although, the above information is consistent with the view of the existence of a genetic basis in endometriosis, other factors could explain the endogenous impact of the disease. Symptomatic women, for example, may seek medical help sooner if they have a relative diagnosed with endometriosis.

According to a study conducted by the Australian National Commission on Health and Social Research on 3,096 twin sisters, endometriosis was observed in 2% of singletons and 0.6% of twins. The increasing incidence of endometriosis in monozygotic twin sisters makes genetic factors more important in the etiology of the disease [29, 30].

5. Diagnosis

When the vaginal bleeding and pelvic pain, which consist symptoms of endometriosis are mild to moderate, the first line treatment is hormonal therapy. Depending on the diagnostic method that will be used, the diagnosis of endometriosis is stated only in 19–20% of cases. The majority of specialists use laparoscopy to diagnose endometriosis. This technique, however, is not without disadvantages. Laparoscopy will diagnose endometriosis in 20% of patients. Another problem with laparoscopy is that even if there are visible lesions, histological confirmation of endometriosis is not always possible. Histological confirmation also depends on the biopsy. In addition, to this due to different forms of the disease, it can be overestimated in more than 2/3 of the patients. Although, is helpful as it allows the patient and clinician to refocus on alternative medical strategies for management, especially in early stages (deep endometriosis). When positive findings – then laparoscopic ablation/resection can be undertaken. The appropriate treatment of endometriosis is of great importance in this age group due to the fact that that fertility should be maintained, also in cases in which tubes are not affected by endometrial lesions because in these cases could be negative laparoscopy findings but could affect fertility(negative influence of occurred endometrial lesions in ovum and sperm). Symptoms of endometriosis are as following: dysmenorrhea 60–80%, pelvic pain 30–50%, subfertility 30–40%, dyspareunia 25–40%, menstrual abnormalities 10–20%, periodical dysuria and hematuria 1–2%, constipation 1–2% and < 1% rectal bleeding and fatigue.

Another big problem for the diagnosis of CPP is that 80% of the patients who have had a laparoscopy has negative findings. And what about these patients who have negative findings? Doyle reports that of the patients with the negative findings, 53% wanted analgesics, 50% were unsatisfied with the treatment and 43% did not have a good quality of life. The presence of endometrial implants in the peritoneum can cause local peritoneal inflammation [30–34].

The cystic form of ovarian endometriosis is usually followed by adhesions, which is known that play an important role in the progression of the disease, explaining why ovarian endometriosis is classified as Π AFS. The determination of Ca-125 is a useful and reliable diagnostic tool, as well as intrarectal ultrasound, while transvaginal ultrasound and magnetic resonance imaging (NMR) are not diagnostic methods used in the diagnosis. Donnez et al. distinguish 3 forms of the disease, endometrial septal endometriosis (Type I), posterior atrial dome endometriosis (Type II) and deep endometrial edema (Type III endometriosis). **Table 1** Koninckx and Martin report another stage of the disease **Table 2**, **Figures 1–5**.

Additional data on the genetic basis of endometriosis, based on sibling studies, are provided by the finding that siblings, non-twins who develop the disease, usually develop the pain symptom at the same age. The incidence of all stages of endometriosis in the sisters of afflicted women in comparison to the general population is six to nine times.

The relationship between endometriosis and increased estrogen production is a popular and biologically plausible hypothesis. Endometriosis and fibroids develop in women of childbearing potential and regress after menopause or after ovulation, which is consistent with the view that the development of these diseases is estrogen dependent.

The estrogen receptor (ER) and the aromatase gene (CYP19) are potential candidate genes. Both could enhance estrogen accumulation and produce a more abundant [34–36].

Thus, it has been investigated whether the polymorphism of the estrogen receptor gene Pa (ER-α) is associated with the development of endometriosis. It is recognized that ectopic endometrial foci have estrogen receptors. Endometrial foci also express cytochrome P450 aromatase, an enzyme that catalyzes the conversion of androgens to estrogens, recommending that local estrogen production may be increased.

Types	Location	Clinical characteristics
Type I	between the posterior vaginal wall and the anterior wall of the muscular wall of the rectum	<2 cm, and most of the lesions are exophytic
Type II	extends from the posterior vaginal septum to the rectal septum	lesions are mostly small and no extension is observed in the orthopedic septum or in the rectal wall
Type III	always located below the parietal peritoneum	infiltration of the muscular wall of the rectum is observed

Table 1.
Distinction of endometriosis according to Donnez et al.

Types	Location	Clinical characteristics	Percentage
Type I	conical shape, infiltration of the surrounding tissues	large pelvic area of endometrial lesions, which are surrounded by off-white connective tissue	4,1%(women with infertility) 10,4% (women with CPP)
Type II	clinically perceived by the diving of the bowel around a typical endometrial lesion	the result of traction of the superficial bowel	0,8%(women with infertility) 3,2%(women with CPP)
Type III	spherical endometrial nodule	most severe form, and often extends laterally around the uterine artery and the corresponding ureter	0,9%(women with infertility) 3,2%(women with CPP)

Table 2.
Distinction of endometriosis according to Koninckx and Martin.

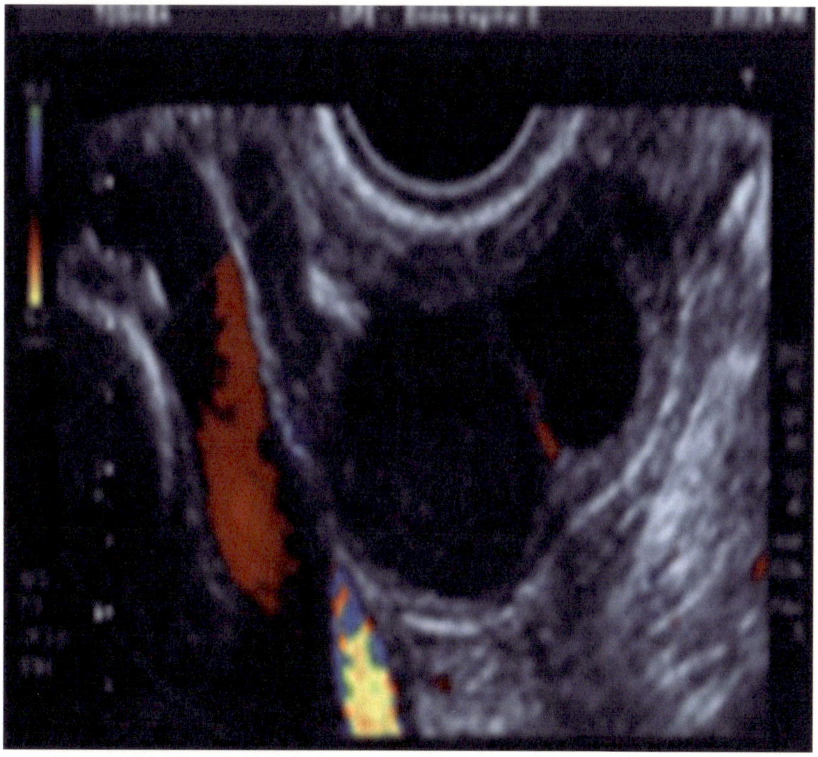

Figure 1.
Ultrasound image showing large endometriomas.

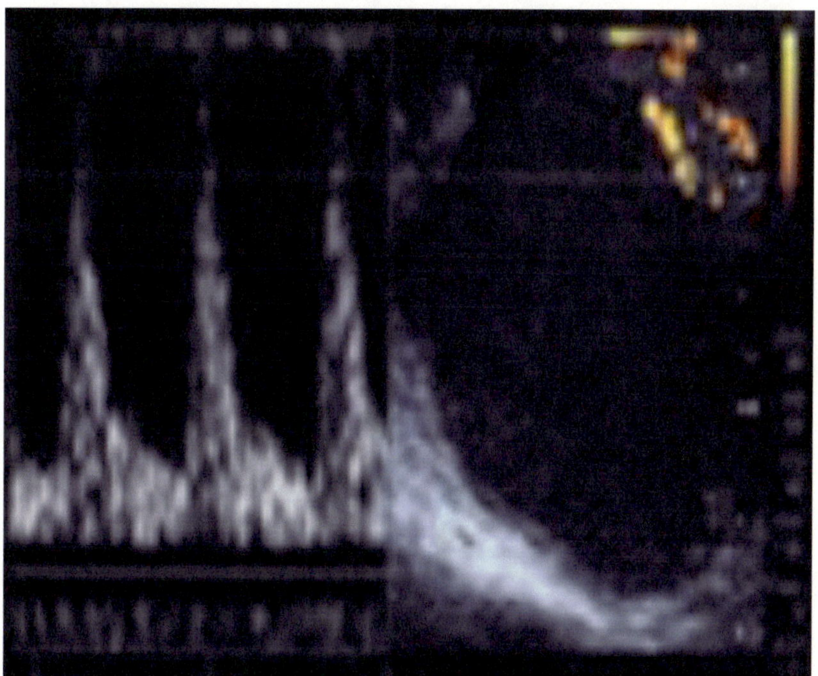

Figure 2.
Doppler ultrasound in endometriomas with high PI (pulsatility index).

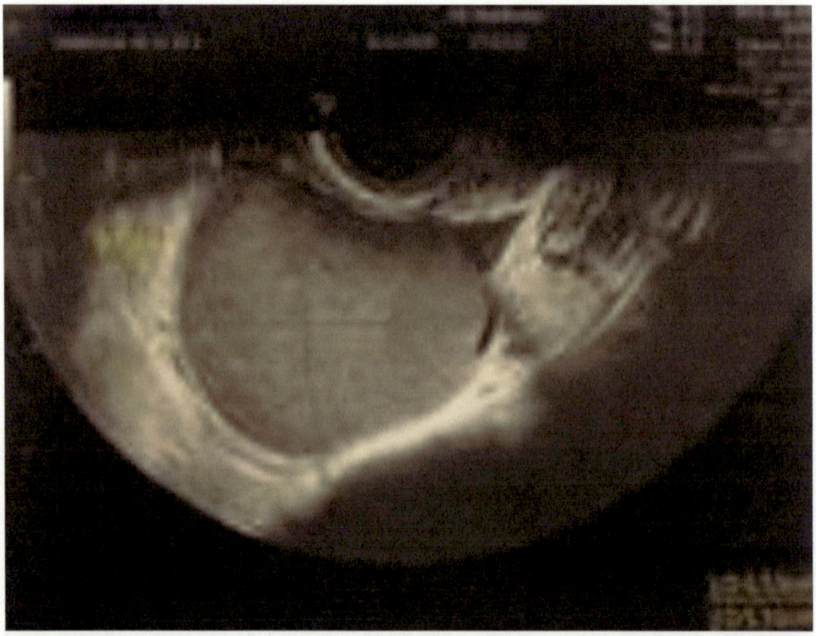

Figure 3.
Ultrasound image of endometriomas (chocolate cyst).

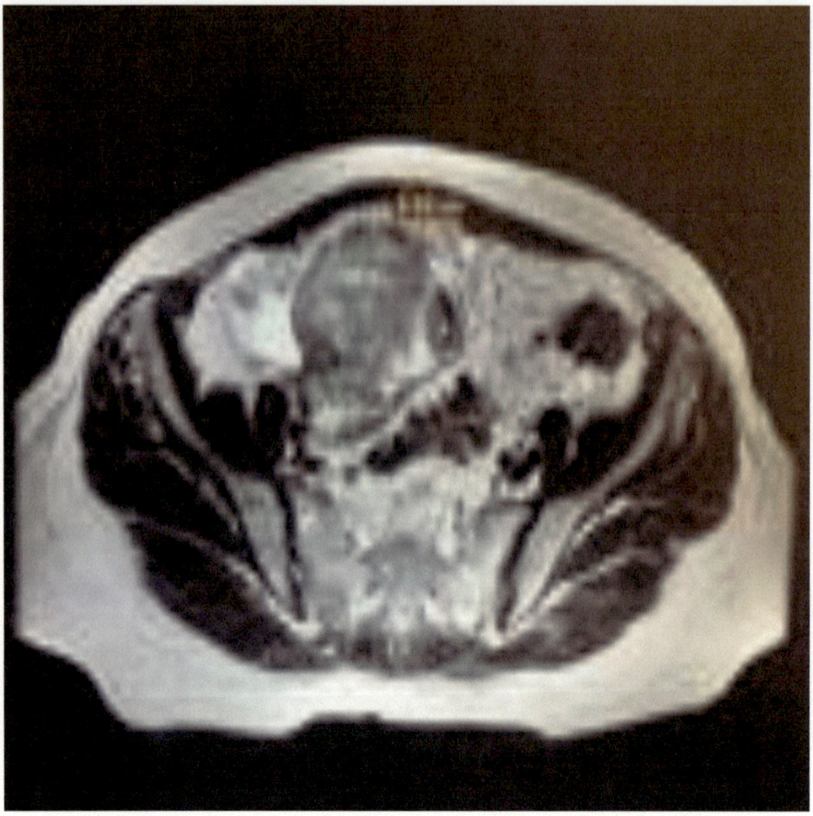

Figure 4.
Pelvic MRI scan showing large endometriomas in cross section.

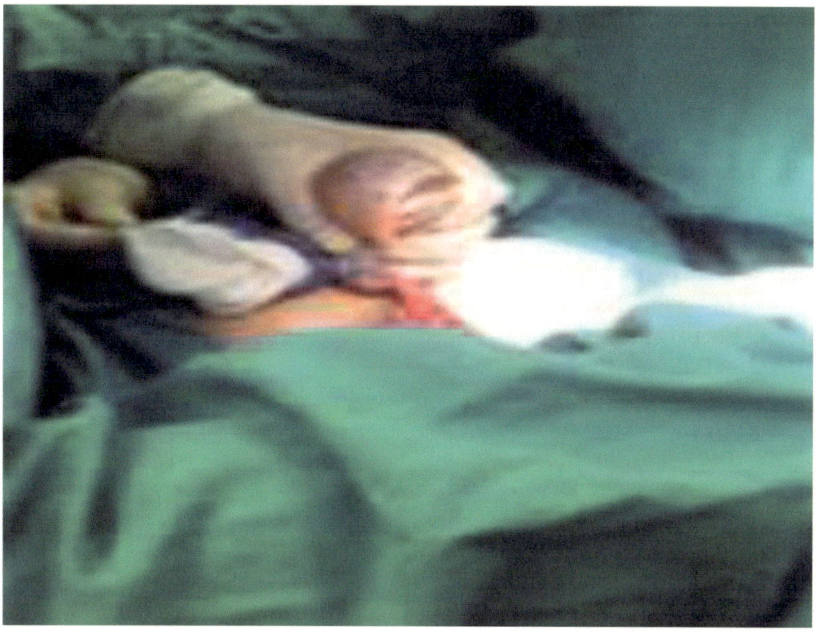

Figure 5.
Ovarian cyst during laparotomy due to ovarian torsion.

Thus, topical estrogens, together with those originating from the bloodstream, stimulate the development of endometrial foci through the estrogen receptor [37–39].

The main support for the action of aromatase in endometriosis is adrenal and ovarian androstenedione. Aromatase converts androstenedione to estrone, a weak estrogen, which must be converted to estradiol to exert a strong eff. In contrast, the enzyme 17β-hydroxysteroid dehydrogenase type II (17β-HSDIII), encoded by a different gene, inactivates estradiol by catalyzing its conversion to conversion by conversion etc.). The enzyme 17β-hydroxysteroid in endometriosis. Progesterone induces the activity of the enzyme 17β-HSDIII in endometrial cell cultures. Expression of 17β-HSD type II is absent from endometrial glandular cells during the secretory phase [37–39].

Moreover, in healthy women PP genotype was less common than PP and Pp genotype, compared with control group women and women with endometriosis. The distribution of genotypes to women in the control group was intermediate between women with endometriosis and women without disease. The frequency of the heterozygous Pp genotype did not differ between the groups. The p allele was less common than the P allele in women without the disease, compared with women with endometriosis and women in the control group from the general population. Thus, PvuII polymorphism of the ER gene is associated with the risk of developing endometriosis. The mechanism by which anonymous intron polymorphism affects the function of the estrogen receptor has not been clarified.

In the future, the clarification of this mechanism will contribute to the understanding of the pathogenesis and pathophysiology of estrogen-dependent diseases of the uterus. Loss of genetic material or DNA refers to loss of heterozygosity. Loss of heterozygosity can be caused by exogenous factors, such as carcinogens which can cause genetic damage that leads to deletions and mutations in DNA [34–39].

Mutations and deletions are particularly important in the remaining tumor suppressor genes, because if one is deleted or inactivated due to a mutation, the gene does not work properly. Such deletions can cause genetic mutations, which lead to inactivation of genes resulting in the loss of heterozygosity. That is, the loss of heterozygosity is the result of the deletion of an area of a putative tumor suppressor gene, leading to the inactivation of that gene. Tumor suppressor genes are altered in ovarian cancers, which is consistent with the view that inactivation of these genes may play a role in the development of endometriosis. LoH heterozygous allelic mutation has been shown to occur for several DNA repair genes MSH2, MSH6, MLH1, and PMS1. The finding of LOH in regions 2p22.3-p16.1 and 3p24.2-p22, where the hMSH2 and hMLH1 genes are located, leads to the hypothesis that in some of the cases of endometriosis there may be a predisposition to cancer. Other evidence suggests the involvement of PTEN, hMLH1, p16 and INK41 in the malignancy of endometriosis. Mutation in hMLH1 methylation has been observed in four of 46 (8.6%) cases of stage III/IV endometriosis. No detectable protein expression of hMLH1 was present in these four cases, the carcinoma coexisted in two, while abnormal methylation of p16 was observed in only one case and reduced protein expression of PTEN was detected in 21 cases (15%). Both of these cases also showed hypermethylation of hMLH.

5.1 Tumor suppressor genes for endometriosis (TP53, PTEN)

Cell monoclonal expression has already been identified in endometriosis by overexpression of certain oncogenic genes (c-myc, c-erg B1). Cytogenetic abnormalities are common in malignancies. Obata and Hoshiai studied: (a) the determination of the cloning of endometriosis foci, (b) the presence of mutations in the TP53 and RASK genes, (c) the lack of heterozygosity at the sites of ovarian cancer, and (d) in endometrial carcinoma. These authors showed a lack of heterozygosity on chromosomes 9p (18%), 11q (18%) and 22q (15%). Overall, 28% of endometriosis foci showed a lack of heterozygosity at one or more sites [33–39].

There is a view that two or more genes are sequentially needed to cause endometriosis. Unlike neoplasms, not all genes involved in endometriosis need to be oncogenes or tumor suppressor genes. We believe that the first "hit" involves a gene that manifests a growing predisposition to attach and implant retrograde menstrual tissue [33–39].

This gene includes the cytoskeleton (MMPs), the cell adhesion molecule (ICAM1)), or macrophage accumulation. The second gene (`hit') may include genes that support endometrial growth, such as the estrogen receptor (ER) or steroid perturbations (CYP19). We also assume that the additional shocks involve a tumor suppressor gene, which leads to uncontrolled cell proliferation. If a tumor suppressor gene is involved in endometriosis, LoH heterozygosity could be lost at such a genetic locus. Iang et al. found the loss of LoH heterozygosity in endometriosis, by studying the chromosomal regions at 9p, 11q, and 22q in endometrial tissue. In a second study, chromosomal alterations were observed in nine of the 11 cases in which ovarian carcinoma had occurred within, or adjacent to, endometriosis [33–39].

Changes in chromosomal regions 5q, 6q, 9p, 11q, and 22q were observed in 25 - -30% of cancer-associated endometriosis cases. This is consistent with the view of some deletion in the areas where the supposed tumor suppressor genes are present, a condition seen in ovarian cancer that coexists with endometriosis. No lack of heterozygosity was found in the normal endometrium. The normal endometrium does not show molecular genetic damage. Tissue samples from endometriosis, adjacent to endometrial carcinoma, atypical endometriosis and endometrial carcinoma of the ovary were examined and common genetic changes were found with stability and joint [33–39].

These common changes did not exist in foci that were far apart. In endometrial cancers, an increased incidence of mutations in the PTEN/MMAC tumor suppressor genes were observed, while no corresponding mutations were found in serous carcinomas and clear cell carcinomas, which is evident for the tumor [33–39].

A second tumor suppressor gene studied in endometriosis is PTEN, which is located on chromosome 10q23. The gene is perturbed in a variety of cancers, including autosomal dominant disorders (Cowden syndrome and Bannayan-Zonana syndrome). PTEN mutations have been reported in endometrial cancers and in an epithelial ovarian tumor, which show some association with endometriosis but not with the serous or mucous epithelial tumors of the ovaries. Mutations involving PTEN have been observed only in endometrial tumors, at 21%. %Sato et al. [33–39] found that LoH heterozygosity was lost for PTEN in eight of 19 endometrial carcinomas (42.1%), in six of 22 clear-cell carcinomas (27.3%), and in 13 of the 23 endometrial cysts. The relationship was even greater when endometrial carcinomas were synonymous with endometriosis [33–39]

Mutations of TP53, PTEN could be associated with the transformation of benign endometrial cells into malignant cells.

In conclusion, in endometriosis there is significant damage to the molecules and to somatic cells. Also, in a percentage of cases, the lesion can continue the progression of the disease. Moreover, regions with chromosomal losses may contain important tumor suppressor genes for the pathogenesis of the disease. Lastly, in a very small percentage of cases, the disease develops into endometrial carcinoma.

6. Abdominal discomfort and pregnancy

In particular, abdominal pain during pregnancy is a the most common phenomenon due to hyperemia of the pelvic vessels or dilation of the ligaments. Due to the frequent occurrence of abdominal pain during pregnancy, it is possible not to diagnose early or even possible pathological causes of abdominal pain.

Fortunately, it is not always associated with a potential risk to pregnancy or to a woman's health, due to pelvic vascular hyperemia or dilation of the round ligaments.

The purpose of this report is to describe some areas of abdominal pain that are less troubling, which of course should be appreciated, and others that dictate immediate medical attention.

Abdominal discomfort should be associated with either a pregnancy complication or a pregnancy-related acute condition. Sometimes after the second trimester, palpable uterine contractions occasionally are painful and frequent in pregnancy.

The diagnosis of childbirth presupposes the existence of rhythmic contractions of a completely eliminated cervix and dilation of the cervix.

Physiological causes of abdominal pain in pregnancy:

Delivery.
Ectopic Pregnancy.
Ovarian cysts.
Uterine torsion.
Preeclampsia.
Placental abruption.
Acid fatty liver in pregnancy.
Musculoskeletal Pain 20–30% of women refer experience lumbar pain and sacroiliac pain.
Natural gases and bloating.

It is very likely that you will have pain caused by gas during pregnancy, due to hormones that slow down the digestion and increasing pressure of the uterus on stomach and intestines.

6.1 Constipation

Sexual intercourse remains one of most common causes of abdominal pain during pregnancy. It is known that the sperm contains prostaglandins, which can "activate" the uterus in some way after ejaculation in the vagina and cause its gentle contractions, which become even more noticeable after orgasm [40–42].

Another point, which means that abdominal pain does not seem to be associated with a serious problem, is its change depending on whether the abdominal pain decreases as soon as gas is released. Rather it is associated with a common and annoying phenomenon, which occurs during pregnancy -: bloating and constipation.

However, there are signs, which, combined with abdominal pain, during pregnancy, are a kind of "alarm" and need immediate investigation:

First of all, if 5 or more uterine contractions occur within an hour, then there is a possibility that premature birth is imminent and it is necessary to administer tocolytic treatment [40–42].

The combination of abdominal pain and vaginal bleeding at any stage of pregnancy is a point of concern. Vaginal bleeding of intense red color, in combination with abdominal pain, depending on the stage of pregnancy during which is, is a point that can hide, miscarriage, premature birth, ectopic pregnancy or placental abruption.

Finally, any abdominal pain during pregnancy, which is very intense, needs to be investigated immediately, because it may be associated with pathology of each of these pregnancies or with pathology independent of pregnancy, which needs immediate treatment. In fact, if this pain is associated with severe nausea and vomiting or fever, it may hide conditions such as appendicitis, nephrolithiasis or cholecystitis [40–42].

7. Treatment of endometriosis and pain

The treatment can be: 1) surgical, 2) conservative.

8. Conservative pharmaceutical treatment

In traditional laparoscopic surgery the percentage of recurrences or non-improvement of symptoms is about 40%. Regarding the corresponding rate of conservative drug treatment, in a study by Waller and Shaw in patients receiving GnRH for 6 months, 30% of patients reported no improvement.

Medical doctors in the field of CPP usually use analgesics or non-steroidal anti-inflammatory drugs or oral contraceptives or progesterone, but have not diagnosed endometriosis from the beginning.

The treatment that has been introduced and is considered as the second line, is GnRH analogues, usually after laparoscopy.

According to the American College of Obstetricians and Gynecologists, the treatment with GnRH analogues is an appropriate approach to failed diagnosis of the cause of pelvic pain [33–39].

9. Traditional surgery treatment

The traditional surgical treatment consists of destruction of the removal of the lesions from the ectopic endometrial tissue, mainly laparoscopically.

If the problem is more dysmenorrhea, there is a high probability of lesions related to the uterine ligaments. In this case, the destruction of the ectopic localized endometrial tissue in the uterosacral ligaments laser can be used.

Also, the cross-section of the uterosacral ligaments with bipolar diathermy has been used.

There are 3 different types of ovarian endometriosis [25].

1. Superficial hemorrhagic lesions

2. Bleeding lesions (endometriomas)

3. Deep ovarian endometriosis

1. In superficial lesions, endometriosis occurs with small cystic lesions in the ovarian cortex or small implants on the lateral surface of the ovary.

2. In endometriomas, the inner surface of a chocolate bladder is essentially the outer surface of the ovary. The hemorrhagic contents of a chocolate bladder can come from a chronic localized hemorrhage, from congested blood vessels, rather than from endometrial apoptosis.

3. In deep ovarian endometriosis there are active endometrial glands that infiltrate the ovarian cortex.

Laparoscopic treatment of ovarian endometriosis includes the following options:

1. Drainage

   The chocolate cyst is aspirated and the cyst cavity is flushed. Postoperatively, subcutaneous injection of GnRH analogues (e.g. goserelin, etc.) is recommended at 0, 4, 8, and 12 weeks [25].

2. Ablation

a. Ovarian endometriomas smaller than 3 cm in diameter treated during the diagnostic laparoscopy, if the cyst is not infiltrated into the ovary to a depth of more than 3 cm, and if the diameter of the cyst is not larger than 3 cm.

   Foci of endometriosis smaller than 1 cm in diameter can be ablated, while endometriomas of 1-3 cm in size are treated as follows: In the beginning, an area is removed from the top of the cyst, the chocolate fluid is aspirated, the ovarian cyst is flushed, and is performed ovarian cystoscopy. Subsequently the inner wall of the cyst is ablated with CO2 Laser at 40 W, until the epithelial layer is damaged (Donnez technique) [25]. However, cauterization of the inner wall of the bladder can be done with monopolar diathermy, endocoagulation or Ultracision as well.

10. Laparoscopic surgery IN CASE the ovarian torsion

Ovarian endometriomas larger than 3 cm in diameter. The protocol proposed by Donnez and applied is the following:

During the diagnostic laparoscopy, a biopsy of the endometrium is taken, the area is rinsed, and then a GnRH analog is administered for 3 months.

A second laparoscopy is performed, and, if the bladder is less than 3 cm, it is ablated as previously described. If the diameter is larger than 3 cm, a part of the cyst is removed (partial ovarian cystectomy) and the ablation of the residual endometroid ovarian cyst is followed.

10.1 Ovarian cystectomy

Described by Semm. The contents of the ovarian cyst are first aspirated, followed by an ovarian cystoscopy of its inner surface. Then, by the guidance/assistance of 2 pairs of contraction forceps, the cyst wall is detached from the ovarian tissue by rotating movements of the forceps that have captured the ovarian cyst wall, and with a movement opposite to the other forceps that has the opposite forceps.

If the ovarian cyst is firmly attached to the area of the ovary, after the remaining part of the ovary has been removed in the manner described above, the part of the ovarian cyst that is firmly attached the ovary may be exposed to CO2.

10.2 Fenestration and ablation

Fayez and Vogel argued that the removal of only one part of the endometrium, in combination with the laser ablation of the remaining part of the ovarian cyst, is associated with the development of fewer adhesions compared to the total removal of the ovarian cyst.

Absence of a thickened capsule around the endometrium makes it difficult to exclude the ovarian cyst wall, resulting in the loss of healthy ovarian tissue during ovarian cystectomy.

Thus, the exclusion of the endometrium through a Fenestration removal of 2 cm of the bladder wall and destruction of the endometrium, appears as the best therapeutic method of surgery on the ovary and the best on the ovary.

Laser laparoscopic treatment, according to Sutton's work, relieved symptoms in 71% of patients after 6 months - while 29% had no improvement. In the same study, one year after laparoscopic treatment, 56% of patients were symptom-free, while 14% had not improved or had relapsed [25, 40–45].

10.3 Additional surgical procedures to treat endometriosis

It has been shown that medication does not cure endometriosis, but makes it temporarily inactive, and that's seems to be the reason of the recurrence after discontinuation of the treatment. Various surgical approaches have been described, such as the use of the CO2 laser in relation to tissue separation and the use of bipolar diathermy.

The use of high-power CO2 laser in superpulse mode has the advantage of accurate tissue cross-section and the simultaneous achievement of hemostasis. On the contrary, the large area of thermal damage after electrocautery makes this approach less accurate, while the clear separation between healthy and abnormal tissue is more difficult. The evolution of the endoscopic equipment, which has been achieved during the last decade, as well the acquired experience and knowledge, have as a result the expansion of the indications of the laparoscopic surgery. The laparoscopic approach is an alternative to laparotomy, which is accompanied by clear and undeniable advantages. However, given that the resection of deep endometriosis is technically extremely difficult and requires vast experience, it is addressed to very few endoscopists. In addition, there are no prospective randomized trials comparing the laparoscopic approach to laparotomy [46].

Laparoscopic surgery is performed by the method of triple puncture, while, when a CO2 laser is used, the surgical laparoscope is angular 12 mm for the diode of the laser beam that is inserted through.

The surgical technique involves separating the anterior surface of the rectum from the posterior surface of the vagina and cutting or sublimating the endometriosis. First, a complete and thorough separation of the anterior surface of the rectum is performed throughout the incision, until the loose tissue of the rectal space appears.

During this surgical step the endometrial catheter is pushed downwards in order to anteriorly inflate the uterus, while some endoscopes use water for separate the fluid from the uterus. After complete preparation, it is cut from the point of adhesion to the rectum. In cases of large infiltration of the vaginal wall, it is necessary to remove part of this vagina, but also the en bloc laparoscopic removal of the entire area followed by closure of the posterior wall of the vagina. In cases of significant degree of infiltration, partial resection of the intestine and final peritoneal anastomosis laparoscopically have been described. The anterior surface of the rectosigmoid junction after surgery is not lubricated, while Interceed can be used to cover the area to be removed. Also, the excision of the intestinal part is restored laparoscopically [46].

Candiani et al. report a decrease in dyspareunia and dysmenorrhea to 60% and 40% after 3.5 years. Candiani et al. also report partial - complete remission of chronic pelvic pain in 70% of patients and a recurrence rate of 5% in 5 years [47].

The pharmaceutical approach to pelvic pain with GnRH analogues also seems to be very adequate. However, the effectiveness of laparoscopic treatment is consider as the first line therapy.

11. Conclusion

The treatment of patients with endometriosis and chronic pelvic pain (COPD) is one of the most challenging situations in every day clinical gynecology medical practice. Chronic pelvic pain is a "key point" for a woman's quality of life.

Nowadays, the diagnosis of the endometriosis still remains difficult despite the knowledge we have acquired after years of study and research. Based on the above there is strong evidence, which supports the position that the pathogenesis of endometriosis is multifactorial, and is influenced by the interaction of genetic and environmental factors. The notion that endometriosis occurs in women with reduced immune function, which is related to genetic predisposition or environmental factors, seems more acceptable in the last decade.

The analysis of the biochemical function of the gene products will lead to a better understanding of the pathophysiology and etiology of endometriosis. New genetic markers can be used to identify high-risk women.

However, the design of epidemiological studies for predisposing factors of endometriosis is insufficient in terms of sample size and phenotype.

Basic research has laid the groundwork for new treatment protocols, particularly useful in women of childbearing age, as understanding pathology is helpful in designing a new improved but permanent treatment.

Acknowledgements

I would like to acknowledge warmest Professor George Iatrakis for supporting this research.

Author details

Panagiotis Tsikouras[1*], Christos Tsalikidis[2], Xanthoula Anthoulaki[1], Anna Chalkidou[1], Aggeliki Gerede[1], Stefanos Zervoudis[3,4], Anastasia Bothou[1], Spyridon Michalopoulos[1], Georgios Dragoutsos[1], Nikolaos Panagiotopoulos[1], Fotini Gaitatzi[1], Ionnis Tsirkas[1], Irini Babgeorgaka[1], Theopi Nalbanti[1], Natalia Sachnova[1], Alexios Alexiou[1], Constantinos Nikolettos[1], Sebaidin Perente[2], Panagiotis Peitsidis[4] and Nikolaos Nikolettos[1]

1 Department of Obstetrics and Gynecology, Democritus University of Thrace Medical School, Alexandroupoli, Greece

2 Second Department of Surgery, Democritus University of Thrace Medical School, Alexandroupoli, Greece

3 Technological Educational Institute of Athens, Athens, Greece

4 Rea Maternity Hospital, Athens, Greece

*Address all correspondence to: tsikouraspanagiotis@gmail.com

References

[1] Zondervan KT, Yudkin PL, Vessey MP, Dawes MG, Barlow DH, Kennedy SH. Patterns of diagnosis and referral in women consulting for chronic pelvic pain in UK primary care. Br J Obstet Gynaecol 1999, 106:1156.

[2] Speer LM, Mushkbar S, Erbele T. Chronic Pelvic Pain in Women. Review Am Fam Physician 2016, 93:380-387.

[3] Daniilidis A, Chatzistamatiou K, Assimakopoulos E. Is there a role for single-port laparoscopy in the treatment of endometriosis? Review Minerva Ginecol 2017, 69:488-503

[4] Powell J. The approach to chronic pelvic pain in the adolescent. Obstet Gynecol Clin North Am. 2014 Sep;41(3):343-55. doi: 10.1016/j.ogc.2014.06.001. PMID: 25155117 Review.

[5] Powell JK. Benign adnexal masses in the adolescent. Adolesc Med Clin. 2004 Oct;15(3):535-47. doi: 10.1016/j.admecli.2004.06.008. PMID: 15625992 Review. Management of chronic pelvic pain. Benjamin-Pratt AR, Howard FM. Minerva Ginecol. 2010 Oct;62(5):447-65. PMID: 20938429 Review.

[6] Stein SL. Gastroenterol Chronic pelvic pain. Clin North Am. 2013 Dec;42(4):785-800. doi: 10.1016/j.gtc.2013.08.005. Epub 2013 Oct 23. PMID: 24280400 Review.

[7] Stewart KA, Parshad-Asnani M, Wonkam A, Bollinger J, Ngo Bitoungui V, Wonkam-Tingang E, et al. "Pain is Subjective": A Mixed-Methods Study of Provider Attitudes and Practices Regarding Pain Management in Sickle Cell Disease Across Three Countries. J Pain Symptom Manage. 2020 Sep 1:S0885-3924(20)30715-6. doi: 10.1016/j.jpainsymman.2020.08.029. Online ahead of print. PMID: 32889040

[8] Benjamin-Pratt AR, Howard FM. Management of chronic pelvic pain. Minerva Ginecol. 2010 Oct;62(5):447-65. PMID: 20938429 Review.

[9] Song AH, Advincula AP. Adolescent chronic pelvic pain. J Pediatr Adolesc Gynecol. 2005 Dec;18(6):371-7. doi: 10.1016/j.jpag.2005.09.001. PMID: 16338601 Review.

[10] Bordman R, Jackson B. Below the belt: approach to chronic pelvic pain. Can Fam Physician. 2006 Dec;52(12):1556-1562. PMID: 17279236

[11] Abduljabbar HS, Bukhari YA, Al Hachim EG, Alshour GS, Amer AA, Shaikhoon MM, Khojah MI. Review of 244 cases of ovarian cysts. Saudi Med J. 2015 Jul;36(7):834-8. doi: 10.15537/smj.2015.7.11690. PMID: 26108588

[12] Moen M. Hysterectomy for Benign Conditions of the Uterus: Total Abdominal Hysterectomy. Obstet Gynecol Clin North Am. 2016 Sep;43(3):431-40. doi: 10.1016/j.ogc.2016.04.003. PMID: 27521877 Review.

[13] Byrnes JN, Trabuco EC. Evidence Basis for Hysterectomy. Obstet Gynecol Clin North Am. 2016 Sep;43(3):495-515. doi: 10.1016/j.ogc.2016.04.009. PMID: 27521881 Review.

[14] Hecht S, Meissnitzer M, Forstner R Acute Pelvic pain in women-gynecological causes. Radiologe. 2019 Feb;59(2):126-132. doi: 10.1007/s00117-018-0475-4. PMID: 30519765 German.

[15] Kruszka PS, Kruszka SJ. Evaluation of acute pelvic pain in women. Am Fam Physician. 2010 Jul 15;82(2):141-7. PMID: 20642266 Review.

[16] Bhavsar AK, Gelner EJ, Shorma T. Common Questions About the Evaluation of Acute Pelvic Pain.

Am Fam Physician. 2016 Jan 1;93(1): 41-48. PMID: 26760839

[17] Kurt S, Uyar I, Demirtaş Ö, Celikel E, Beyan E, Tasyurt A. Acute pelvic pain: evaluation of 503 cases. Arch Iran Med. 2013 Jul;16(7):397-400. PMID: 23808776

[18] Winkel CA. Role of a symptom-based algorithmic approach to chronic pelvic pain. Int J Gynaecol Obstet. 2001 Sep;74 Suppl 1:S15-S20. PMID: 11549395

[19] Barker MA. Current Issues with Hysterectomy. Obstet Gynecol Clin North Am. 2016 Sep;43(3):591-601. doi: 10.1016/j.ogc.2016.04.012. PMID: 27521886 Review.

[20] Stratton P, Sinaii N, Segars J, Koziol D, Wesley R, Zimmer C, Winkel C, Nieman LK. Return of chronic pelvic pain from endometriosis after raloxifene treatment: a randomized controlled trial. Obstet Gynecol. 2008 Jan;111(1):88-96. doi: 10.1097/01.AOG.0000297307.35024.b5. PMID: 18165396

[21] Gambone JC, Mittman BS, Munro MG, Scialli AR, Winkel CA.; Consensus statement for the management of chronic pelvic pain and endometriosis: proceedings of an expert-panel consensus process. Chronic Pelvic Pain/Endometriosis Working Group. Fertil Steril. 2002 Nov;78(5):961-972. doi: 10.1016/s0015-0282(02)04216-4. PMID: 12413979

[22] Winkel CA. Modeling of medical and surgical treatment costs of chronic pelvic pain: new paradigms for making clinical decisions. Am J Manag Care. 1999 May;5(5 Suppl):S276-S290. PMID: 10537662

[23] 23.M Brigid Holloran-Schwartz 1 . Surgical evaluation and treatment of the patient with chronic pelvic pain Obstet Gynecol Clin North Am 2014 Sep;41(3):357-369. doi: 10.1016/j.ogc.2014.05.003. Epub 2014 Jul 14.

[24] Szamatowicz M. Gynecol Endometriosis--still an enigmatic disease. What are the causes, how to diagnose it and how to treat successfully? Endocrinol. 2008 Oct;24(10):535-6. doi: 10.1080/09513590802296062. PMID: 19012093 No abstract available.

[25] Baldi A, Campioni M, Signorile PG. .Endometriosis: pathogenesis, diagnosis, therapy and association with cancer (review). Oncol Rep. 2008 Apr;19(4): 843-6. PMID: 18357365 Review.

[26] Donnez J. Introduction: From pathogenesis to therapy, deep endometriosis remains a source of controversy. Fertil Steril. 2017 Dec;108(6):869-871. doi: 10.1016/j.fertnstert.2017.10.015. PMID: 29202962

[27] Doyle JO, Missmer SA, Laufer MR. The effect of combined surgical-medical intervention on the progression of endometriosis in an adolescent and young adult population. J Pediatr Adolesc Gynecol. 2009 Aug;22(4):257-263. doi: 10.1016/j.jpag.2008.11.003. PMID: 19646673

[28] Donnez O, Roman H. Deep endometriosis: definition, diagnosis, and treatment. Fertil Steril. 2017 Dec;108(6):931-942. doi: 10.1016/j.fertnstert.2017.09.006. PMID: 29202966 Review.

[29] Donnez J. Endometriosis: enigmatic in the pathogenesis and controversial in its therapy. Fertil Steril. 2012 Sep;98(3):509-510. doi: 10.1016/j.fertnstert.2012.07.1125. PMID: 22938767

[30] Azarani A, Osias J, Berker B, Nezhat C, Nezhat C. Endometriosis: insights into its pathogenesis and treatment. Surg Technol Int. 2004;12:178-81. PMID: 15455323 Review.

[31] I. Stavrou, C. Zois, J.P.A. Ioannidis, A. Tsatsoulis. Association of polymorphisms of the oestrogen receptor α gene with the age of menarche Human Reproduction, Volume 17, Issue 4, April 2002, Pages 1101-1105, https://doi.org/10.1093/humrep/17.4.1101

[32] Sundarrajan, C,., Liao, W.X., Roy AC,, A.C. and Ng SC, S.C. Association between estrogen receptor-beta gene polymorphisms and ovulatory dysfunction in patients with menstrual disorders. J. Clin. Endocrinol. Metab. 86, 135-139. 2001

[33] Guo SW. Nuclear factor-kappab (NF-kappaB): an unsuspected major culprit in the pathogenesis of endometriosis that is still at large?. Gynecol Obstet Invest. 2007;63(2):71-97. doi: 10.1159/000096047. Epub 2006 Oct 4. PMID: 17028437 Review.

[34] Riemma G, Laganà AS, Schiattarella A, Garzon S, Cobellis L, Autiero R, Licciardi F, Della Corte L, La Verde M, De Franciscis P. Ion Channels in The Pathogenesis of Endometriosis: A Cutting-Edge Point of View. . Int J Mol Sci. 2020 Feb 7;21(3):1114. doi: 10.3390/ijms21031114. PMID: 32046116

[35] Flyckt R, Kim S, Falcone T. Surgical Management of Endometriosis in Patients with Chronic Pelvic Pain. Semin Reprod Med. 2017 Jan;35(1): 54-64. doi: 10.1055/s-0036-1597306. Epub 2017 Jan 3. PMID: 28049215 Review.

[36] Yeung PP Jr, Shwayder J, Pasic RP. Laparoscopic management of endometriosis: comprehensive review of best evidence. J Minim Invasive Gynecol. 2009 May-Jun;16(3):269-81. doi: 10.1016/j.jmig.2009.02.007. PMID: 19423059 Review

[37] Donnez J, Pirard C, Smets M, Jadoul P, Squifflet J. Surgical management of endometriosis. Best Pract Res Clin Obstet Gynaecol. 2004 Apr;18(2):329-48. doi: 10.1016/j.bpobgyn.2004.03.004. PMID: 15157646 Review.

[38] Donnez J, Donnez O, Dolmans MM. Introduction: Uterine adenomyosis, another enigmatic disease of our time. Fertil Steril. 2018 Mar;109(3):369-370. doi: 10.1016/j.fertnstert.2018.01.035. Epub 2018 Mar 8. PMID: 29526476

[39] Donnez J, Van Langendonckt A. Typical and subtle atypical presentations of endometriosis. Curr Opin Obstet Gynecol. 2004 Oct;16(5):431-7. doi: 10.1097/00001703-200410000-00013. PMID: 15353954 Review.

[40] Zeng C, Xu JN, Zhou Y, Zhou YF, Zhu SN, Xue Q. Reproductive performance after surgery for endometriosis: predictive value of the revised American Fertility Society classification and the endometriosis fertility index. Gynecol Obstet Invest. 2014;77(3):180-185. doi: 10.1159/000358390. Epub 2014 Mar 1. PMID: 24603632

[41] Maheux-Lacroix S, Nesbitt-Hawes E, Deans R, Won H, Budden A, Adamson D, Abbott JA. Endometriosis fertility index predicts live births following surgical resection of moderate and severe endometriosis. Hum Reprod. 2017 Nov 1;32(11):2243-2249. doi: 10.1093/humrep/dex291. PMID: 29040471

[42] Koninckx PR, Zupi E, Martin DC. Endometriosis and pregnancy outcome. Fertil Steril. 2018 Aug;110(3):406-407. doi: 10.1016/j.fertnstert.2018.06.029. PMID: 30098688

[43] Donnez J, Squifflet J, Donnez O. Minimally invasive gynecologic procedures. Curr Opin Obstet Gynecol. 2011 Aug;23(4):289-95. doi: 10.1097/GCO.0b013e328348a283. PMID: 21666466 Review.

[44] Nisolle55Nisolle M, Donnez J. Peritoneal endometriosis, ovarian endometriosis, and adenomyotic nodules of the rectovaginal septum are three different entities. Fertil Steril. 1997 Oct;68(4):585-96. doi: 10.1016/s0015-0282(97)00191-x. PMID: 9341595 Review.

[45] When more is not better: 10 'don'ts' in endometriosis management. An ETIC (*) position statement. ETIC Endometriosis Treatment Italian Club. Hum Reprod Open. 2019 Jun 12;2019(3):hoz009. doi: 10.1093/hropen/hoz009. eCollection 2019. PMID: 31206037

[46] Donnez J, Squifflet J, Pirard C, Jadoul P, Wyns C, Smets M. The efficacy of medical and surgical treatment of endometriosis-associated infertility and pelvic pain. Gynecol Obstet Invest. 2002;54 Suppl 1:2-7; discussion 7-10. doi: 10.1159/000066288. PMID: 12441654 Review.

[47] Candiani M. .Current guidelines for treatment of endometriosis without laparoscopy. Drugs Today (Barc). 2005 Jul;41 Suppl A:11-5. PMID: 16200220

Chapter 4

Hysteroscopy, the Window into the Uterine Cavity

Shani Naor-Revel, Ruth Goldstone and Ariel Revel

Abstract

Hysteroscopy, is a technique by which we can look into the uterine cavity entering through the cervix and is today the most applied minimally invasive technique in Gynecology. Indications for hysteroscopy include infertility investigation, abnormal uterine bleeding, and evaluation of suspicious sonographic findings. Nowadays we approach the uterus via vaginoscopy with no anesthetic. Once inside the uterus, we remove polyps or stringless IUD and take a biopsy. These procedures are often referred as "see and treat". Operative hysteroscopy under GA or sometimes cervical block, uses larger instruments to resect myomas, cut a septum (metroplasty) or separate intrauterine adhesions (Asherman's). As Glycine is no more used in hysteroscopy it has become quite a safe procedure. Use of disposable scopes will enable this tool to be part of every gynecologic clinic.

Keywords: hysteroscopy, infertility, uterine bleeding, menorrhagia, metrorrhagia, intrauterine device, septate uterus, asherman's uterine adhesion, fibroids, endometrium, polyps, see and treat

1. Introduction

In 1950, doctors could expect medical knowledge to double every 50 years. By 2020, it will take just 73 days. How's a doctor supposed to keep up? [1]. Writing a chapter to a textbook is thus a challenge. Even if we succeed in being up to date by the time this chapter is published it might already be obsolete. The reader should thus read the chapter as an introduction and follow up on the topics read. As carrying out hysteroscopies requires manual training, we hope that the gynecologist reading our chapter will gain theoretical understanding along with his or her training first on a simulator before performing this procedure on real patients. We think that a gynecology resident should perform 100 diagnostic hysteroscopy procedures before attempting an operative one.

2. History of hysteroscopy

"Hysteroscopy" comes from the Greek terms hysteros meaning uterus and scopy meaning to look. Hysteroscopy enabled visualization of a narrow and dark space, which was difficult until the mid-nineteenth century. Endoscopy was invented by Bozzini in 1805. The first successful hysteroscopy however was performed 65 years later by Pantaleoni when he investigated the uterus of a 60-year-old patient complaining of postmenopausal bleeding. Bozzini detected a polyp in the uterus which

Nitze	1877	Magnifying lense
Heineberg	1914	Parallel chanel, continuous flow
Rubin	1925	CO2 insufflation
Mickulicz-Radecki	1927	electrocoagulation
Vulmiere	1952	Fiber optics
Harold Horace Hopkins and Storz	1959	Rod lens optic
Marleschki	1965	contact hysteroscope
Edström and Fernström	1970	Dextran
Hamou	1980	Glycine
Bettochi	1997	Office scope

Table 1.
Milestones in the development of the hysteroscope.

he cauterized with silver nitrate. Bozzini died at 35 years of age from typhoid fever, and his attempts to improve the light conductor ended. **Table 1** mentions some of the pioneers that have contributed to the hysteroscope.

For distending the uterine cavity for operative hysteroscopy normal saline is used nowadays as it is significantly less dangerous than glycine when fluid loss occurs. Hysteroscopy today represents 200 years of significant innovations in instrumentation, new clinical applications for existing instruments, and continual modification of techniques, all aiming at observing, diagnosing, and treating pathologic conditions of the uterine cavity.

3. Indications

Indications for diagnostic hysteroscopy include many conditions where knowledge about the endometrial cavity is relevant to patient care but the scope of this chapter has not been able to go into depth for every indication. In **Table 2** we list the most common indications for the procedure as well as which tools are required and how long we recommend for such a procedure. This may help the team communicate with each other and referring physicians and the patients, where should the procedure be scheduled and how long it should take and which equipment is required for the procedure.

3.1 Menstrual cycle bleeding

Bleeding at menstruation (menorrhagia) or in between them (metrorrhagia). Postmenopausal bleeding should include a blind biopsy. Patients with bleeding under hormonal replacement therapy should be examined. A frequent referral are patients on continuous Tamoxifen therapy [2]. Bleeding under medical therapy requires a pathological sampling to exclude malignancy. Pipelle ® sampling has 100% sensitivity and specificity to detect malignant cells [3].

Heavy menstrual bleeding is a significant health problem in pre and perimenopausal women. If no pathology is diagnosed using diagnostic hysteroscopy and biopsy, patients should be counseled about treatment which could be hormonal and non-hormonal. As medical therapy is not always successful, Endometrial ablation may be an alternative to hysterectomy that preserves the uterus. Many techniques have been developed to ablate the endometrium. First-generation techniques require visualization of the uterus with a hysteroscope during the procedure.

		Inpatient/ outpatient	Additional Instruments needed	Estimated procedure time (minutes)
10.1	Menorrhagia/ Metrorrhagia/ bleeding under medical therapy	Out	Pipelle ®	3
10.2	Products of conception	In	Grasper/loop	10–30
10.3	Failed clinics attempt to remove IUD/parts	Out	Grasper	5
10.4	abnormal/thick/echoic endometrium by sonography	Out	Pipelle ®	3
10.5	Asherman's	In	Needle tip	10–50
10.6	Fibroid/ metroplasty	In	Loop	5–50
10.7	Primary/secondary infertility and assessing tubal patency	Out	Bubbles sometimes Pipelle ®	5
10.8	Habitual abortions	Out	Pipelle ®	3
10.9	Niche	In	Loop	5–15

Table 2.
Inpatient or outpatient indications for hysteroscopy, device and time needed to complete the procedure.

Second- and third-generation techniques are quicker than previous approaches because they do not require hysteroscopic visualization during the procedure. Decision as to visual or blind procedure is based on the skills of the surgeon and on the size of the uterus. Results and patient satisfaction appear to be similar [4].

3.2 Postpartum or post miscarriage/induced abortion bleeding

Postpartum bleeding raises a suspicion of placental remains. There also may be bleeding due to retained products of conception following an abortion either spontaneous or induced for medical reasons.

3.3 IUD related

Common referral to hysteroscopy is to remove an IUD. In cases where the strings are not apparent referral to hysteroscopy is preferable to the patient than attempting blind instrument IUD extraction.

3.4 Suspected malignancy by sonography

Often the indication is sonographic findings such as suspicion of submucosal uterine fibroids, adenomyosis, endometrial cancer. It should be stressed that following removal of a polyp and diagnosis of malignancy it is obligatory to plan hysterectomy even if the rest of the cavity seemed normal in hysteroscopy. In an Israeli study, residual complex atypical hyperplasia (CAH) or endometrial cancer (EC) was present in 89% of the hysterectomy specimens, mostly (55.6%) as multifocal lesions [5].

3.5 Asherman's

Hysteroscopy is currently considered the gold standard diagnostic and therapeutic approach for patients with intrauterine adhesions [6]. An integrated approach, including preoperative, intraoperative, and postoperative therapeutic measures, however, are warranted owing to the complexity of the syndrome.

3.6 Fibroid, septate uterus

Hysteroscopic removal of endometrial polyps suspected on ultrasound in women prior to IUI and IVF may improve the clinical pregnancy rate compared to simple diagnostic hysteroscopy [6].

3.7 Primary/secondary infertility; assessing tubal patency

Hysteroscopy should be part of evaluation of primary and secondary infertility [6]. The performer should investigate and describe the uterine shape to exclude a septate uterus or other Mullerian abnormalities of the uterus, the endometrium to exclude intrauterine synechia (adhesions, Asherman's) and atrophy. Moreover an attempt to pass bubbles via the tubal ostia determines tubal patency [7].

3.8 Habitual abortions/recurrent pregnancy loss (RPL)

When a woman has 3 or more consecutive spontaneous abortions we recommend evaluation which includes a diagnostic procedure to evaluate the uterine cavity. Office hysteroscopy, is the easiest and most informative tool to investigate possible intrauterine abnormalities such as septate uterus or intrauterine adhesions or a polyp in patients with RPL or recurrent implantation failure (RIF).

3.9 Niche

Control examination of the uterine cavity after operations on the uterus such as cesarean to see the niche, curettage to evaluate whether there are remains, Asherman's to evaluate the reappearance of adhesions. Following metroplasty for septate uterus it is good practice to evaluate the cavity by hysteroscopy to confirm if postoperatively the uterine cavity is fit for pregnancy. In some cases, a reoperation is required to complete cutting an extensive septum. Also, following myomectomy it is recommended to repeat hysteroscopy to judge whether there are any remnants of the myoma and that no postoperative adhesions have formed.

4. The hysteroscopy team

The hysteroscopy clinic enables patients to undergo the procedure in the office setting. Patients can continue their day plans without need to cancel pleasure activities or work. The team involves administrative, nursing and the physician. It is quite important for the team to work in a concerted way so that the patient arrives at the correct time and the correct equipment is ready for the procedure.

4.1 The administrative assistant

An experienced secretary is an important player for a well-orchestrated team to work coherently. When a patient calls in for an appointment, you should transfer the call to a dedicated secretary and follow a planned call questionnaire. The most important question is asking about the date of the patient's last menstrual period. In premenopausal women, hysteroscopy should be performed between days 7–11 following the beginning of the menstrual period. This achieves a certainty about our patient not being pregnant and the lining of the uterus is thin, in order to see a good view of the uterus. The patient is advised to eat before coming to the clinic to reduce the complication of a low blood sugar or weakness after the procedure.

In case of doubt the patient is required to carry out βhCG in the blood before coming the clinic. if this was not performed, a urinary pregnancy test to ensure βhCG is negative. Moreover, it is easier to introduce the scope during menstruation as the cervix is slightly relaxed.

4.2 Nursing

Dedicated and professional nursing is an integral part of hysteroscopy. We find it quite efficient to have three nurses working with the physician hysteroscopist in the diagnostic and in the see and treat hysteroscopy clinic. One nurse sits with the patient and explains to her the procedure and prepares her for the signing of the informed consent with the physician and to offer the patient oral analgesia before the procedure.

The second nurse will be assisting the physician during the procedure making sure that the equipment is sterile, connecting the light cable and the normal saline to the scope as well as handing over surgical tools such as grasper or scissors to perform a 'see and treat' procedure and to ensure the wellbeing of the patient. The patient will be seated and covered by the nurse and at the end of the procedure the nurse will ensure that the patient safely descends from the gynecological chair and is able to go and get dressed on her own.

The third nurse oversees sterilization of the hysteroscope optics and sheaths.

It is recommended for a busy clinic to have quite a few both diagnostic and 'see and treat' scopes. We usually schedule a dozen patients per clinic morning, sterilization must thus be carried out in parallel to performing the procedures so that unprepared equipment is not the bottleneck of the clinic. It is recommended that the hysteroscopy clinic nurse attends courses given to physicians or to nurses about hysteroscopy, its indications, contraindications and how the procedures are performed. Teaching a new nurse should be done by an experienced nurse to ensure that safety and efficacy are carried out. Only after such training should a new nurse assist a hysteroscopy clinic. In the UK, a nurse hysteroscopist performs diagnostic procedures [8]. In Israel and to the best of our knowledge in mainland Europe and North America however, only physicians are licensed to carry out invasive procedures on live patients.

Before signing the informed consent, the nurse briefs the patient on the hysteroscopic procedure. Main points explained are the following:

- The hysteroscope is inserted through the vagina and cervix into the uterus. It is very fine and ordinarily a speculum is not used.

- Liquid solution is passed through the hysteroscope throughout the procedure, to expand the uterus and to clear away any blood or mucus.

- The physician will gently insert the hysteroscope which has a light source and can also introduce small tools through a side port. This will enable her to have also a treatment such as removing a polyp or an intrauterine device.

- The nurse explains to the patient that she must read the consent form before sitting with the doctor and any questions regarding the consent form she will be able to receive an explanation before the procedure from the doctor.

4.3 The Gynecologic surgeon

A hysteroscopist is usually a certified gynecologic surgeon. There is mounting evidence in the surgical literature to support the use of skilled labs outside of the operating room for resident training and indeed simulation is the key point for an appropriate surgical learning [9]. It is necessary to improve the quality of the simulators by enhancing or introducing tactile feedback [10].

The physician must carry out three main duties prior to beginning hysteroscopy.

Firstly, review the patient's medical, gynecological, and obstetrical history in general and the reason for referral to the procedure.

Secondly, explain the indication to the patient and thus discuss expectations. For example, if it is to evaluate the endometrial cavity prior to embryo transfer, or to remove an IUD. Another example is suspicion of postpartum residual placental tissue where it should be clear that we will need to schedule an operative procedure as the amount of tissue to be removed exceeds possibility by see and treat equipment.

Thirdly the physician is responsible to rule out an ongoing pregnancy. In case of any suspicion, the patient performs a urinary or blood hCG.

It is imperative that the doctor detail and explain the very rare complications of a procedure prior to starting surgery. The physician should make sure the patient understands that there are rare complications in less than 1% of cases. Anesthesia if used, has rare complications. Intrauterine infection is a contraindication for hysteroscopy. Perforation of the uterus can occur and should be diagnosed immediately by the gynecologist. In such complication the patient will be evaluated to rule out possible damage to her bowel, blood vessel or bladder. Intrauterine adhesions may occur following operative surgery, especially for large lesion such as a myomectomy. With the use of normal saline as distending medium there are no adverse reaction to the distention media as was seen sometimes with Glycine or Dextran. After reviewing such these rare complications, the physician and patient are now ready to sign an informed consent form.

5. The equipment

Equipment that is needed to perform diagnostic hysteroscopy includes the fibreoptic scope, a light cable, and the camera. The camera is connected to a screen. It is recommended to have a camera and a printer to capture and then insert pictures into your operative report. Through an operating channel mechanical tools can be inserted to carry out a 'see and treat' procedure in an outpatient setting [11]. Moreover, the advent of new technologies is further changing the approach of outpatient hysteroscopic surgery. Some procedures that in the past required cervical dilatation to introduce the resectoscope can currently be perfomed using a thin hysteroscope [12].

For all purposes we use a 1.9 (2.8 with sheath) millimeter rigid hysteroscope. For the see and treat the diameter is 4.2 millimeter with the scope of 2.9 millimeter. We find those scopes are well tolerated even by nulliparous or postmenopausal patients.

5.1 Distension of the uterine cavity

Currently we use normal saline for all our hysteroscopic procedures. The use of Glycine is dangerous as it may cause hyponatremia [13]. For the diagnostic procedure the one- or three-liter bag of normal saline flows using gravity is used. It is however easier to use a balloon handpump as sometimes the patient has blood clots in the uterine cavity that need to be flushed out so the gynecologist can see the endometrial cavity.

5.2 Single use scopes

Clinics commonly perform hysteroscopy with multiple use equipment. Recently single use hysteroscopes have been developed (Neoscope or Lina operascope). This may be a suitable option at a gynecologist office where few procedures are performed.

5.3 Hysteroscopy tissue removal systems

Hysteroscopic tissue removal systems (Truclear®, Myosure® or IBS®) may offer an advantage in successful removal of pathology and shorten total operation time.

6. Hysteroscopic method

For purpose of clarity, we will describe how to perform outpatient and inpatient procedures, separately.

6.1 Outpatient hysteroscopy

In order to overcome the sensation of pain caused by speculum and tennaculum among patients undergoing office hysteroscopy the vaginoscopy approach (no touch) was first proposed by Bettocchi [14]. The method uses no insertion of speculum nor any instruments to grasp the uterine cervix. The performer uses vocal analgesia. This means that you keep talking to your patient while performing the procedure and not necessarily showing her the instruments that you use. The patient is encouraged to look at the screen and be part of the procedure. In a randomized trial, oral analgesia was shown to reduce pain [15].

The patient is covered in lithotomy position with her legs comfortably in stirrups. There is no need for scrubbing nor washing. Following digital gentle separation of the major labia and gently inserting the tip of the hysteroscope, the performers eyes are then reverted to the screen while filling the vagina with normal saline.

At this point the cervix should be located. Usually, the uterine cervix will be found in the posterior part of the vagina, you then direct the scope to the opening of the cervix and gently land on it with your scope in order to enter. The rigid hysteroscope needs to gently enter into the cervical canal. The scope has a 30 degree angle and therefore while going through the cervical canal the opening of the canal should be seen at 6 o'clock and gently slide along the cervical canal until the inner os of the uterine cavity is observed. In a retroverted uterus this is the opposite, the hands should be reversed and therefore the opening of the cervix will be seen at 12 o'clock. When the uterus is very introverted you could use your hand to put a little suprapubic pressure on the uterus in order to straighten it. You can use one hand at this step in order to enter the uterus and if needed ask a nurse to apply the suprapubic pressure or even the patient herself. The entry to the uterine cavity should be performed very slowly and carefully watching in order to prevent pain and in order to avoid the possibility of entering forcefully and causing a perforation. Throughout the procedure the patient should be relaxed. The physician should perform all actions slowly using the left hand to hold the camera in a fixed position while the scope with a 30 degree angle is moved along the longitudinal axis, observing the right wall then the anterior wall, then the left wall and then the posterior wall. All these should be done by rotating the attachment of the light cable to the hysteroscope, Taking pictures is recommended.

The whole procedure is performed very slowly., retracting the scope looking on the exit at the lower anterior wall of the uterus. This is especially relevant in patients who had a previous cesarean section, in order to observe if there is a niche. Looking at the cervical canal can give some information about the possibility of a polyp. The instrument is then removed from the vagina. The whole procedure should take no longer than one minute.

6.2 See and treat

Performance of diagnostic and operative procedures for gynecological conditions in the consultation room setting is becoming increasingly commonplace to reduce risks of general anesthetic, decrease healthcare costs and increase convenience for both patient and gynecologist. Diagnostic hysteroscopy is performed using the required instrument (e.g. scissors or grasper) on standby inside the working canal. Intrauterine contraceptive device (IUD) removal or its fragments is a common referral. Use of small diameter hysteroscopes and resectoscopes allow these procedures to be performed as a single stage "see-and-treat" hysteroscopy in the comfort and safety of an office-based setting.

6.3 Operative

Hysteroscopic surgery has become the standard of care to treat benign intrauterine disease in pre-menopausal and even postmenopausal women. The various hysteroscopic procedures have been shown as safe and highly effective to treat lesions such as submucous myomas, endometrial polyps, uterine septa and intracavitary adhesions.

Operative hysteroscopy is performed in the OR and thus offers advantages and disadvantages. Advantages include the possibility to remove large pathologies from the uterine wall. The operative hysteroscope is inserted following dilatation of the uterine cervix to hegar dilator 10-10.5 under general anesthesia.

There are 3 parts to the operative procedure. First the dilatation of the cervix. This might turn out to be the risky part and indeed most complications occur at this step [6]. The second part deals with the pathology, whether it be using the loop to resect a polyp or type 0 submucosal fibroid [pedunculated fibroids without any intramural extension]. It is more difficult to remove a type 1 [submucosal with minor intramural] fibroid. Type 2 fibroids [mostly intramural, the angle with the endometrium is>90°] should not be removed by hysteroscopic surgery.

7. Analgesia

With new hysteroscopes, it is possible not only to examine the cervical canal and uterine cavity but also to perform biopsies or treat benign diseases in a relatively short time, without any premedication for anesthesia. This is because the sensory innervation of the uterus mainly regards the myometrium, while the endometrium and the fibrous tissue of septa and synechiae are almost insensative [16]. Preventing pain is very important.The pain is caused by distending the uterus and mostly in the cervical canal.

7.1 Analgetics

The use of rectal indomethacin, ropivacaine or levobupicavaine diluted in the saline distension medium, the use of multimodal local anesthesia as well as the use of premedication by means of diclofenac potassium or tramadol are all effective methods to reduce pain. There is a lack of consensus on the choice of analgesia for outpatient hysteroscopy, with a recent meta-analysis and systematic review suggesting oral nonsteroidal anti-inflammatory drugs and transcutaneous electrical nerve stimulation (TENS) for pain relief [17].

7.2 Preparation of the cervix with vaginal misoprostol

Giving low-dose (25 mcg) Misoprostol before the procedure may soften the cervix sufficiently to allow an easier and more successful test. This medication has been tested before intrauterine procedures including hysteroscopy and, in some patients, it has been shown to be beneficial. Cervical priming facilitated hysteroscopy by dilating the cervix, allowing for easier entry and reducing procedural time. Administration of a cervical preparation, however, increased the risk of adverse effects, namely genital tract bleeding, abdominal pain/cramping and gastrointestinal disturbance [18].

7.3 Distraction techniques

Non-pharmacological options of pain relief at outpatient hysteroscopy include music, hypnosis, adjusting the temperature and pressure of distension medium, stretching of the uterus with a full bladder and electricity via TENS. What we usually do is to have a cheerful conversation with the patient, and we suggest controlled breathing in order to relax the body. It is helpful to suggest to the patient to watch the screen as we explain what we see. Since this chapter is written during the covid-19 pandemic we do not allow the partner to join the patient. Somewhat surprisingly we are under the impression that this has resulted in reducing patient stress.

7.4 Virtual reality

Virtual reality (VR) was suggested as a distraction technique for non-pharmacological pain relief. It is a computer-generated representation of an immersive environment viewed through a headset. VR is effective in reducing pain and anxiety during outpatient hysteroscopy [19].

8. Contraindications

Hysteroscopy is contraindicated in patients with Pelvic infection, Pregnancy, Cervical cancer or Heavy uterine bleeding. If the contraindications to hysteroscopy are observed, complications should be rare.

9. The hysteroscopy reports

The medical report represents one of the most critical steps not only from a legal, medical point of view but also for the patient and other health professionals. It should first include the description of the instruments used: hysteroscope, optics, distension medium, and any mechanical or energy tools. Subsequently, the technique used for access to the cervical canal should be reported, plus the morphology of the cervical canal and the uterine cavity should be carefully described. We report the visualization of both the tubal Ostia and whether they appear patent by passing bubbles. Findings such as polyps, fibroids, adhesions, or a septum should be described in detail. This includes location, size, vascularization, and severity. At the end of the report, your patient should receive recommendations. If surgery is required it should be stated and a referral for surgery added. In patients undergoing infertility treatment it should be added when the exam is normal that the uterus appears to be compatible for pregnancy. This will indicate to the patient and the infertility team that it is recommended to proceed with IVF or other methods used.

Before discharge, all information written in the letter should be explained to the patient and questions should be answered in detail so that the patient has all the information required for further treatment.

10. Complications

Morbidity and even death have been reported after hysteroscopic interventions [20, 21].

10.1 Adhesions resulting in defective endometrial receptivity

Hysteroscopic resection of a polyp, fibroid or placental pregnancy products is frequently performed to increase IVF success rates. Moreover, a septate uterus may hinder pregnancy following embryo transfer. Hysteroscopic adhesiolysis is the gold standard intervention to treat intrauterine adhesions.

Nevertheless, intrauterine procedures by themselves may cause defective endometrial receptivity [22].

We thus carry out the procedure with paramount prudence so as not to harm normal endometrium nor cause adhesions. In patients who have children, it is crucial to know before surgery if the patient has completed her family plans. For example, if a patient in her 40's has perimenopausal menorrhagia is undergoing hysteroscopic polypectomy the operation would be carried out in different mode whether she wants to preserve her fertility potential or not. This should be described in her informed consent. Some have claimed that endometrial thickness is narrower following polypectomy. We have looked into this and have found that our pregnancy rates were higher despite a mild postoperative decrease in endometrial thickness [23].

10.2 Perforation of the uterine wall

The most common complication of hysteroscopy is uterine perforation (approximately 1%) which can occur with a blunt instrument (uterine sound, dilator, curette, hysteroscope) or during the use of an energy source such as electrosurgery (i.e., inappropriate use of electrodes), with a possible injury of the surrounding organs (bladder, bowel, vessel) resulting in catastrophic consequences. An alternative to the utilization of a thermal energy source during hysteroscopic surgery is the use of mechanical energy such as scissors or intrauterine morcellator (IUM) to treat benign pathologies such as polyps, myomas, and retained products of conception.

10.3 Infection

The prevalence of infections following in-office hysteroscopy is low (0.06%) [24]. routine antibiotic prophylaxis is thus unnecessary before hysteroscopy. Patients should be counseled that if they have fever following an hysteroscopic procedure they should contact your office or out of hours go to the gynecology emergency room.

10.4 Bleeding

In most patients, we performed the procedure on the last days of the menstrual cycle therefore bleeding is still present before and after hysteroscopy. The patient should be informed that mild bleeding is normal after the procedure nevertheless if severe bleeding ensues or continues the patient should contact the clinic or out of hours go to the emergency room to exclude a serious complication from the hysteroscopic procedure. In diagnostic hysteroscopy we perform a procedure using the new vaginoscopic approach, therefore in most cases there is no bleeding at all from the procedure itself. In inpatient hysteroscopy. anesthesia we use the tenaculum and Hagars to dilate the cervix, therefore bleeding results mostly from the surgical intervention. Also following the removal of fibroids or polyps some bleeding is expected, although this should stop within a few hours following the procedure. In some cases removing a large fibroid leaves a large area of exposed blood vessels and attempts should be made during the procedure to obtain hemostasis using coagulation. If bleeding continues the physician may introduce an intrauterine Foley catheter and inflate it, which should be removed an hour later. In most cases, this stops the bleeding and patient is discharged home only after evaluation that there is no substantial bleeding after surgery.

11. Cost

In Israel, most procedures are performed in the HMO setting and therefore it is free for our patients. According to the Israeli ministry of health price list the reimbursement for a diagnostic hysteroscopy is 606 NIS whereas, for a surgical procedure the reimbursement is 1,104 NIS.

In USA, the cost of a hysteroscopy ranges from $750-$3,500. The cost depends on the extent of the procedure. For instance, a diagnostic-only procedure is much less than one involving surgery. The cost may be higher for a more extensive procedure which includes surgery in the hospital and general anaesthesia. Costs for these extensive procedures can be up to $7,000. Some US health insurance carriers will cover a hysteroscopy, at least partially.

In an Italian paper [25], total hospital costs for polypectomy with all systems were significantly less expensive in an office setting compared with same-day surgery in the hospital setting ($p = .0001$).

12. Conclusions

Hysteroscopy is an essential part of the gynecologist's toolbox. Nowadays, hysteroscopy is the gold standard for the diagnosis and treatment of intrauterine pathologies as it represents a safe and minimally invasive procedure that allows the visualization of the entire uterine cavity. It is an inexpensive however valuable method. Cervical preparation before examination with vaginal misoprostol reduces pain during outpatient hysteroscopy and can be offered particularly to nulliparous or postmenopausal patients. Hysteroscopy requires certain skills and experience and is not exempt from complications, especially in unexperienced hands. The report should describe the method used to perform the procedure and then the relevant findings. This includes the shape of uterine cavity, the endometrium, and the right and left ostia. In infertile patients, describe whether bubbles travel through the fallopian tube openings. Gynecologist should be familiar with this tool for better evaluation and treatment of their patients.

Acknowledgements

Rabbi Yitchok Melber for kindly reviewing the manuscript.

Conflict of interest

The authors declare no conflict of interest.

Notes/thanks/other declarations

This paper is dedicated in memory of my friend Dr. Yaron Aaron Hamani, MD. A dear friend and a fine gynecologist who passed away at young age.

Author details

Shani Naor-Revel[1*], Ruth Goldstone[2] and Ariel Revel[3]

1 Shamir Medical Center, Affiliated to the Sackler School of Medicine, Tel Aviv University, Tel Aviv, Israel

2 Misgave Ladakh Hospital, Meuhedet HMO, Jerusalem, Israel

3 Division of Reproductive Endocrinology and Infertility, Shamir Medical Center, Affiliated to the Sackler School of Medicine, Tel Aviv University, Tel Aviv, Israel

*Address all correspondence to: shaninaor3@gmail.com

References

[1] Staying Current in Medicine: Advice for New Doctors - NEJM Knowledge+ [Internet]. [cited 2017 Mar 8]. p. undefined-undefined. Available from: https://www.mendeley.com/catalogue/7042e372-504f-302b-bafd-34322b4be523/?utm_source=desktop

[2] Bakkum-Gamez JN, Laughlin SK, Jensen JR, Akogyeram CO, Pruthi S. Challenges in the gynecologic care of premenopausal women with breast cancer. Mayo Clin Proc [Internet]. 2011 Mar [cited 2021 May 29];86(3):229-40. Available from: http://www.ncbi.nlm.nih.gov/pubmed/21307388

[3] Utida GM, Kulak J. Hysteroscopic and aspiration biopsies in the histologic evaluation of the endometrium, a comparative study. Med (United States) [Internet]. 2019 Oct 1 [cited 2021 Feb 10];98(40). Available from: https://pubmed.ncbi.nlm.nih.gov/31577708/

[4] Bofill Rodriguez M, Lethaby A, Fergusson RJ. Endometrial resection and ablation versus hysterectomy for heavy menstrual bleeding. Cochrane Database Syst Rev [Internet]. 2021 Feb 23 [cited 2021 May 7];2021(2). Available from: https://pubmed.ncbi.nlm.nih.gov/33619722/

[5] Elyashiv O, Sagiv R, Kerner R, Keidar R, Menczer J, Levy T. Hysterscopic Resection of Premalignant and Malignant Endometrial Polyps: Is it a Safe Alternative to Hysterectomy? J Minim Invasive Gynecol [Internet]. 2017 Nov 1 [cited 2021 Feb 12];24(7):1200-3. Available from: https://pubmed.ncbi.nlm.nih.gov/28802955/

[6] Wessel van S, BWJ BosteelsJ M, WesselS van. Cochrane Library Cochrane Database of Systematic Reviews Hysteroscopy for treating subfertility associated with suspected major uterine cavity abnormalities (Review) Hysteroscopy for treating subfertility associated with suspected major uterine cavity abnormalities (Review). 2018 [cited 2021 Feb 20]; Available from: www.cochranelibrary.com

[7] Vitale SG, Carugno J, Riemma G, Török P, Cianci S, De Franciscis P, et al. Hysteroscopy for Assessing Fallopian Tubal Obstruction: A Systematic Review and Diagnostic Test Accuracy Meta-analysis. Journal of Minimally Invasive Gynecology. Elsevier B.V.; 2020.

[8] Jones SE. The role of the nurse hysteroscopist. Rev Gynaecol Pract. 2005 Sep 1;5(3):196-9.

[9] Kerbage Y, Rouillès J, Estrade JP, Collinet P, Huchon C, Villefranque V, et al. Surgical training through simulation dedicated to French Ob-gyn residents. Evaluation and satisfaction. J Gynecol Obstet Hum Reprod. 2021 Sep 1;50(7):102076.

[10] Vitale SG, Caruso S, Vitagliano A, Vilos G, Di Gregorio LM, Zizolfi B, et al. The value of virtual reality simulators in hysteroscopy and training capacity: a systematic review. Vol. 29, Minimally Invasive Therapy and Allied Technologies. Taylor and Francis Ltd; 2020. p. 185-93.

[11] Dealberti D, Riboni F, Cosma S, Pisani C, Montella F, Saitta S, et al. Feasibility and Acceptability of Office-Based Polypectomy With a 16F Mini-Resectoscope: A Multicenter Clinical Study. J Minim Invasive Gynecol. 2016 Mar 1;23(3):418-24.

[12] Shveiky D, Rojansky N, Revel A, Benshushan A, Laufer N, Shushan A. Complications of hysteroscopic surgery: "Beyond the learning curve." J Minim Invasive Gynecol. 2007;14(2):218-22.

[13] Manchanda R, Valenti G, Rathore A, Carugno J, Török P, Riemma G, et al. Distension media delivery systems in hysteroscopy: past, present and future [Internet]. Minimally Invasive Therapy and Allied Technologies. Taylor and Francis Ltd; 2020 [cited 2021 Mar 3]. Available from: https://pubmed.ncbi.nlm.nih.gov/32410478/

[14] Bettocchi S, Selvaggi L. A vaginoscopic approach to reduce the pain of office hysteroscopy. J Am Assoc Gynecol Laparosc. 1997 Feb 1;4(2):255-8.

[15] Ogden J, Heinrich M, Potter C, Kent A, Jones S. The impact of viewing a hysteroscopy on a screen on the patient's experience: a randomised trial. BJOG An Int J Obstet Gynaecol [Internet]. 2009 Jan 1 [cited 2021 Feb 28];116(2):286-93. Available from: http://doi.wiley.com/10.1111/j.1471-0528.2008.02035.x

[16] Brauer M. Plasticity in Uterine Innervation: State of the Art. Curr Protein Pept Sci [Internet]. 2016 Dec 14 [cited 2021 Feb 20];18(2):108-19. Available from: http://www.eurekaselect.com/openurl/content.php?genre=article&issn=1389-2037&volume=18&issue=2&spage=108

[17] De Silva PM, Mahmud A, Smith PP, Clark TJ. Analgesia for Office Hysteroscopy: A Systematic Review and Meta-analysis [Internet]. Vol. 27, Journal of Minimally Invasive Gynecology. Elsevier B.V.; 2020 [cited 2021 Feb 12]. p. 1034-47. Available from: https://pubmed.ncbi.nlm.nih.gov/31982584/

[18] De Silva PM, Wilson L, Carnegy A, Smith PP, Clark TJ. Cervical dilatation and preparation prior to outpatient hysteroscopy: a systematic review and meta-analysis [Internet]. BJOG: An International Journal of Obstetrics and Gynaecology. Blackwell Publishing Ltd; 2020 [cited 2021 Feb 12]. p. 1471-0528.16604. Available from: https://onlinelibrary.wiley.com/doi/10.1111/1471-0528.16604

[19] Deo N, Khan K, Mak J, Allotey J, Gonzalez Carreras F, Fusari G, et al. Virtual reality for acute pain in outpatient hysteroscopy: a randomised controlled trial. BJOG An Int J Obstet Gynaecol [Internet]. 2021 Jan 22 [cited 2021 Feb 11];128(1):87-95. Available from: https://onlinelibrary.wiley.com/doi/10.1111/1471-0528.16377

[20] A Scottish audit of hysteroscopic surgery for menorrhagia: complications and follow up. BJOG An Int J Obstet Gynaecol [Internet]. 1995 Mar [cited 2021 Feb 12];102(3):249-54. Available from: http://doi.wiley.com/10.1111/j.1471-0528.1995.tb09103.x

[21] Aydeniz B, Gruber I V., Schauf B, Kurek R, Meyer A, Wallwiener D. A multicenter survey of complications associated with 21 676 operative hysteroscopies. Eur J Obstet Gynecol Reprod Biol. 2002 Sep 10;104(2):160-4.

[22] Revel A. Defective endometrial receptivity. Fertil Steril. 2012 May 1;97(5):1028-32.

[23] Kogan L, Dior U, Chill HH, Karavani G, Revel A, Shushan A, et al. Operative hysteroscopy for treatment of intrauterine pathologies does not interfere with later endometrial development in patients undergoing in vitro fertilization. Arch Gynecol Obstet. 2015;1-4.

[24] Florio P, Nappi L, Mannini L, Pontrelli G, Fimiani R, Casadio P, et al. Prevalence of Infections After In-Office Hysteroscopy in Premenopausal and Postmenopausal Women. J Minim Invasive Gynecol. 2019 May 1;26(4):733-9.

[25] Franchini M, Lippi G, Calzolari S, Giarrè G, Gubbini G, Catena U, et al. Hysteroscopic Endometrial

Polypectomy: Clinical and Economic Data in Decision Making. J Minim Invasive Gynecol [Internet]. 2018 Mar 1 [cited 2021 Mar 5];25(3):418-25. Available from: http://www.jmig.org/article/S1553465017304399/fulltext

Section 3

Minimally Invasive Approaches in Cardio-Thoracic Surgery

Chapter 5

Minimally Invasive Approaches in the Thoracic Surgery

Güntuğ Batıhan and Kenan Can Ceylan

Abstract

Minimally invasive techniques in thoracic surgery have made great progress over the past 20 years and are still evolving. Many surgical procedures performed with large thoracotomy incisions in the past can now be performed with much smaller incisions. With many studies, the advantages of minimally invasive surgery have been clearly seen, and thus its use has become widespread worldwide. Today, minimally invasive surgical methods have become the first choice in the diagnosis and treatment of lung, pleural and mediastinal pathologies. Minimally invasive approaches in thoracic surgery include many different techniques and applications. In this chapter, current minimally invasive techniques in thoracic surgery are discussed and important points are emphasized in the light of the current literature.

Keywords: Lobectomy, minimally invasive surgery, robotic surgery, video-assisted thoracic surgery

1. Introduction

Minimally invasive surgical approaches have become widely used in chest surgery as they are applied in every area of medicine. With the use of smaller incisions and modern instruments, patient comfort has increased, and hospital stays have been shortened.

Due to the rigid structure of the thorax, ventilation of the lung, and the presence of large vascular structures in the mediastinum, it has not been easy to adapt minimally invasive methods to thoracic surgery. While initially limited to simple biopsy procedures and wedge resections, nowadays, extended lung resections can be performed with minimally invasive surgery.

Advantages of thoracoscopic lobectomy compared to thoracotomy include less postoperative pain, better pulmonary function, early recovery, shorter hospitalization have shown by many studies, and Video-assisted thoracic surgery (VATS) has become established as a gold standard treatment method for patients with early-stage lung cancer [1–6].

2. Brief history of lung resections

In human history, wars, traumas and infections have created the necessity for surgical interventions and provoked its development. Lung resection performed by Rolandus in a patient with pulmonary herniation due to trauma in 1499 has taken its place as the first case in the literature. Similarly, Nicholas Tulp surgically treated a patient with herniated lung due to chest trauma. The surgical method he applied was "ligatured it and cut it off with scissors: it weighed three ounces" [7].

Frederik Ruysch (1638–1731) described a case of traumatic lung herniation. He ligated the herniated lung and preformed serial dressing changes until the necrotic lung sloughed off [8].

The first case of resection for a lung tumor was reported in 1861 by Jules Emil Pean. He performed lung resection by suturing the pleura to the lung and, removing it with galvanic current cautery [9].

Lung resections performed until the beginning of the 20th century were based on cutting a portion of the lobe by ligaturing. In 1927 Whittemore presented his exteriorization lobectomy. In this procedure, the lung was firmly sutured to the muscles of the chest wall with deep stitches and the wound closed as tightly as possible. The main logic here is to make the tissue sloughed off by creating gangrene in the part of the lung to be removed [10].

One-staged lobectomy was firstly described by Brunn in 1927. He performed lobectomy in patients with bronchiectasis and used the technique of hilar clamping, ligation, and suturing with phrenicotomy to keep the diaphragm immobile. He also completely closed the pleural cavity and chest wall and used an intercostal catheter for drainage [8, 11, 12].

In the following years, the importance of anatomical dissection of hilar structures was understood and individual ligation and suturing of the anatomical structures were performed in lung resections.

Adapting the innovations in technology to surgical treatment methods started a new era in thoracic surgery.

Lewis et al. reported 100 consecutive VATS lobectomy in 1992. He stapled the hilar structures without individual dissection. The use of this technique has raised suspicion in the surgical community against VATS, and individual isolation and ligation of the hilar structures have continued [13].

The technique of anterior-to-posterior isolation and ligation of the hilar structures was firstly described by McKenna [14]. This approach has been adopted and successfully applied by many surgeons. Even if the port numbers changed, the basic approach remained as the anterior to posterior dissection and division of the hilar structures separately (**Figures 1** and 2).

Many studies conducted in the following years showed the superiority of VATS over thoracotomy in postoperative pain, drainage time, length of hospital stay and postoperative complications [14–16].

With the increasing experience, many thoracic surgery procedures and advanced lung resections can be successfully performed with VATS today. Although

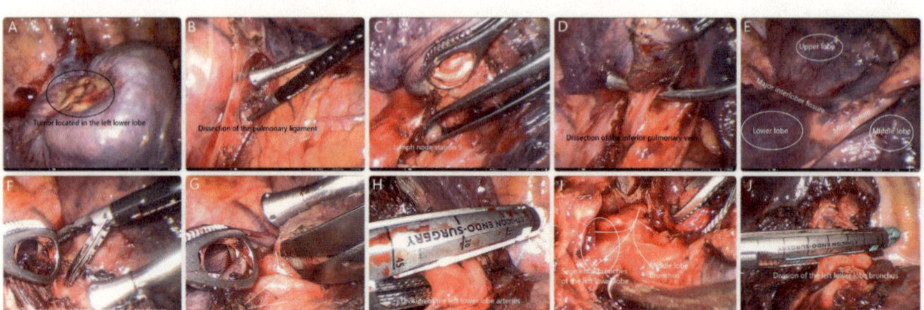

Figure 1.
VATS right lower lobectomy was performed for the lung cancer located in the right lower lobe. Intraoperative photographs of important steps were collaged.

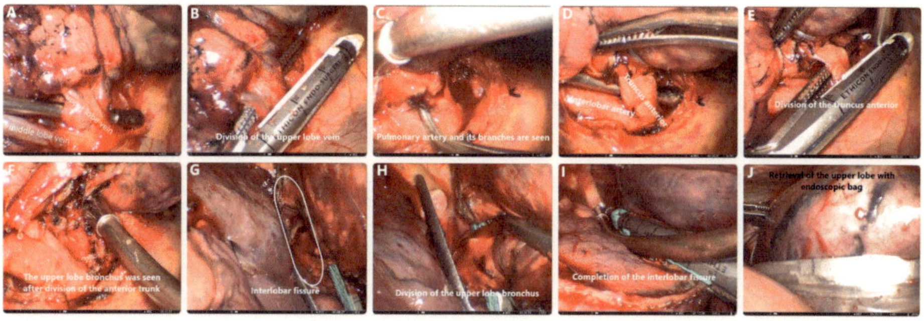

Figure 2.
VATS right upper lobectomy was performed for the lung cancer located in the right upper lobe. Intraoperative photographs of important steps were collaged.

the basic approach remains the same, different techniques have emerged over time in videothoracoscopic surgery. Below, we have tried to summarize different approaches under the heading of surgical techniques.

3. Surgical technique

Due to the nature of thoracic surgery, its relationship with anesthesiologists is more advanced than other surgical specialties. The single-lung ventilation, which may be accomplished with either double-lumen endobronchial tubes or with single-lumen tubes and bronchial blockers, is often required. Placement of a thoracic epidural catheter for postoperative pain control is essential. Therefore, the presence of an experienced anesthesiologist is of great importance for the intraoperative and postoperative process to go smoothly.

The patient is positioned in full lateral decubitus position with slight flexion of the table at the level of the mid-chest, which allows slight splaying of the ribs to

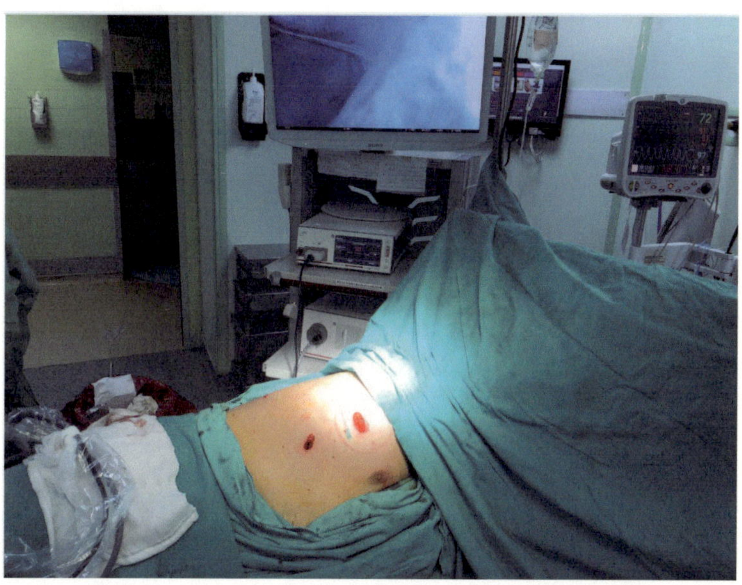

Figure 3.
Patient and camera position during VATS.

improve exposure in the absence of rib spreading. The operator and assistant stand at the front of the patient and the monitor is positioned at the back (**Figure 3**).

Endoscopic instruments like endostaplers, endograspers and dissectors, endoscopic bag and energy devices should be readily available. The number of ports varies depending on the instruments available, the experience of the team and the surgeon's personal preference.

3.1 3-port VATS

In this technique, a 1.5 cm camera port along the midaxillary line is located in the 7th or 8th intercostal space in the midaxillary line. The main access (utility) port was usually placed in the anterior axillary line 4th intercostal space for an upper lobectomy or 5th intercostal space for a lower lobectomy. The posterior port is placed at the level of seventh or eighth intercostal space along the posterior axillary line (**Figure 4**).

The posterior port provides an ideal angle for endoscopic staplers and vascular structures can be divided without difficulty. In addition, when necessary, the camera is moved to the posterior port to make a better exploration and a safe dissection of the hilar structures in the posterior [15, 16].

3.2 2-port VATS

Although there are different variations in this technique in terms of the placement of the camera port, in our clinic, we prefer the middle or anterior axillary

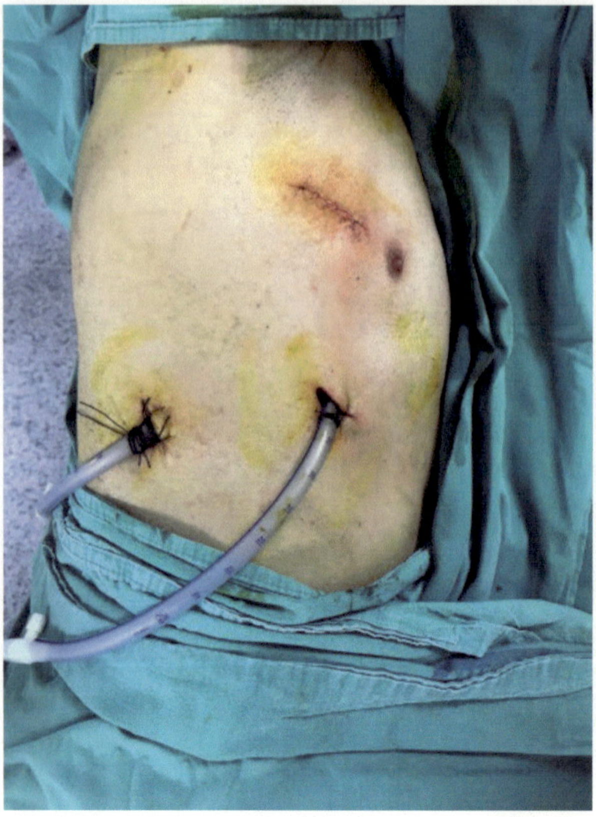

Figure 4.
Incisions in the 3-port VATS technique.

line 7–8. intercostal space. The location of the utility port is similar to the 3-port technique (**Figure 5**).

Due to the lack of a posterior port in this technique appropriate retraction maneuvers must be done to ensure safe dissection. The use of more than one instrument through the anterior port opening to compensate for the absence of the posterior port is not recommended due to the risks of intercostal nerve injury and long-term postoperative pain.

3.3 Uniportal VATS

Surgeons have always been attracted by the notion that surgical procedures can be performed through a single incision. Three-port and bi-portal VATS lobectomy is well established and have been preferred by many thoracic surgeons however with increasing experience, the search for a less invasive technique continued.

Uniportal VATS is firstly described by Dr. Gaetano Rocco in 2004 for minor thoracic procedures include pleural biopsies, sympathectomies, debridements of early-stage empyema. In this study, Rocco stated that wedge resections can be performed successfully as in the classical three-port technique and emphasized the superiority of uniportal surgery [17].

The first uniportal VATS lobectomy was reported by Gonzalez-Rivas in 2011. In the following years, Gonzales demonstrated that even the most complex lung resections can be performed with uniportal VATS successfully and safely. Uniportal VATS has become preferred by many surgeons due to its advantages, such as causing less tissue damage and providing direct vision [18, 19].

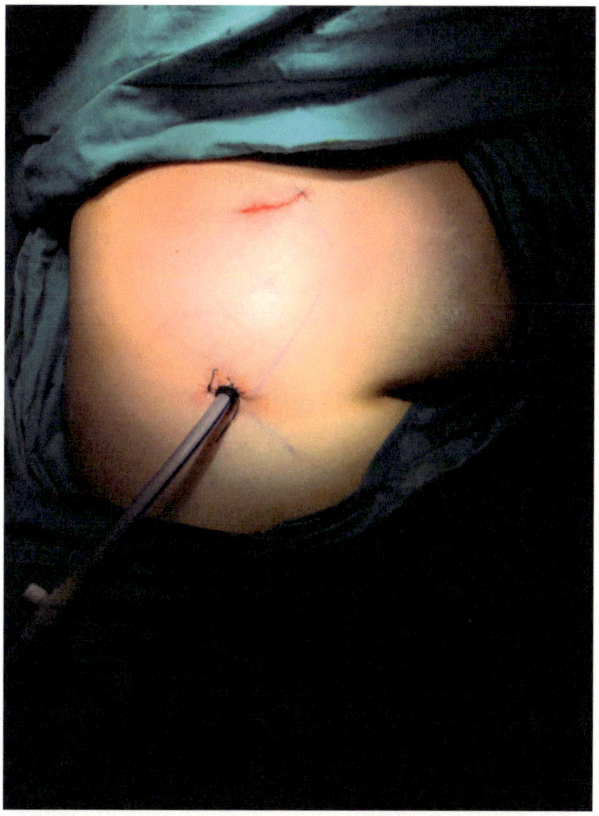

Figure 5.
Incisions in the 2-port VATS technique.

3–5 cm uniport incision is placed in the 5th intercostal in the anterior axillary line. A 5 mm diameter 30° video-thoracoscope is inserted through the same incision Thus, the assistant and the surgeon share the same vision of direction. Although this is beneficial in terms of team cooperation, the working environment of the surgeon is somewhat limited.

3.4 Needlescopic VATS

As the name suggests, Needlescopic VATS is a minimally invasive surgical procedure performed by keeping port incisions as small as possible. The term of "needlescopic", which was first defined for laparoscopy, was later used for VATS [20–22]. General acceptance is that port incisions in needlescopic VATS are smaller than 3 mm and therefore, the essentials of this approach are appropriate equipment and instruments. Using this approach, diagnostic procedures, pneumothorax operations and sympathectomies have been successfully performed. This technique can also be used for lung resections by making a utility incision in addition to the needlescopic ports. Ko HJ et al. reported the results of 75 patients who underwent uniportal and needlescopic VATS anatomic resection and defined needlescopic approach as a bridge between multiport and uniportal thoracic surgery [23, 24].

During the past 15 years at our center, approximately 800 patients have undergone VATS lobectomy. Each of the approaches detailed above has been applied in our clinic, and as a result, the 3-port approach has been adopted more heavily. Our experience has shown that the posterior port provides a very suitable angle for hilar dissection and stapler use, and significantly reduces the operation time. In addition, the lung can be retracted with the grasper used from the posterior port and the operator can work with two hands. Whichever approach is used in VATS, the important thing is to complete the learning curve and to expand the patient scale that can benefit from VATS by increasing experience in the approach used.

With the increasing experience, the patient group with a history of locally advanced lung cancer or neoadjuvant therapy can also benefit from minimally invasive surgery and extended lung resections can be performed successfully.

4. Robot-assisted thoracic surgery (RATS)

The adaptation of the robotic system to the thorax has opened new horizons for thoracic surgeons. Features superior to VATS can be summarized as follows [25–27]:

1. Filtration of physiologic hand tremor

2. Ten times magnification and the 3D high definition camera

3. Thanks to the robotic arms that offer articulation it is easier to perform complex surgical maneuvers, comfortable reach to the narrow spaces.

4. By offering the surgeon an ergonomic position, it reduces the risk of muscle fatigue during the operation.

However, despite all these features, its use has not become widespread due to its high cost, long installation and lack of tactile feedback, but undoubtedly, all surgical procedures will evolve towards robotization in the near future.

5. Diagnostic performance of VATS in thoracic pathologies

Minimally invasive surgical methods have become a good alternative for patients who cannot be diagnosed with non-invasive diagnostic methods. VATS is successfully applied for diagnostic purposes in sampling of mediastinal lymph nodes, undiagnosed mediastinal masses, and parenchymal lesions [28–30].

EBUS-TBNA is a safe and feasible procedure for the diagnosis of mediastinal lymph nodes. However, in mediastinal pathologies, especially in cases where large tissue sampling is required, it is not always possible to diagnose with EBUS. VATS is feasible for mediastinal lymph nodes and tumors with a sensitivity of 100%. VATS is an appropriate method for sampling 5th and 6th station lymph nodes in lung cancer staging, which cannot be reached by either EBUS or mediastinoscopy. Contrary to the alternative methods that can be used for sampling the lymph nodes in this region, VATS can be used to evaluate the thoracic cavity and the T factor of the tumor simultaneously.

VATS is a successful method in the diagnosis of parenchymal nodules as well as mediastinal pathologies. Although non-surgical methods include CT-guided percutaneous needle aspiration and transbronchial biopsy are the first choice in the diagnosis of small pulmonary nodules, the success rate of these methods is low in lesions below 1 cm and subsolid nodules.

Although it is a safe and feasible method, it can be difficult to detect small and subsolid nodules with VATS because of the lack of tactile feedback and of bimanual palpation. Various pre-operative and perioperative marking techniques were described in the literature to facilitate intraoperative detection of small-sized or subsolid nodules [30–32].

Methylene blue, metal wire, micro coil or Technetium-99 can be used for marking the parenchymal nodules [30–33]. Because it is effective, easy to apply and inexpensive, we prefer preoperative CT-guided injection of methylene blue to marking the pulmonary nodules in our clinic. However, an experienced interventional radiologist who has good communication with the surgical team is required for the successful application of this technique.

6. VATS resection in the treatment of lung cancer

The application of VATS lobectomy in the surgical treatment of lung cancer has a history of approximately 30 years. Lewis et al. published the first VATS lobectomy series in the literature, involving 3 patients with lung cancer in 1992. [13]. In 1999, a series of 400 cases were published by the same author [34]. However, the surgical technique used in these studies was far from the modern VATS lobectomy, which involves the dissection of hilar structures separately.

McKenna Jr. described the first VATS lobectomy that forms the basis of today's practice, which includes anatomic dissections with individual ligation of the vessels and bronchi. He and his colleagues reported 1100 cases with NSCLC who underwent VATS lobectomy [14]. Many studies demonstrating the superiority of VATS over thoracotomy followed this study, which presented a short hospital stay, low mortality and morbidity rates.

In the following years, uniportal VATS lobectomy was described by Gonzalez-Rivas. He presented the results of 102 patients who underwent uniportal VATS lobectomy in 2013. In this study mean surgical time was 154.1 ± 46 minutes and the median duration time of a chest tube was 2 days and the median length of hospital stay was 3 days [18, 19]. In the following years, Gonzales Rivas shared his experiences showing that the uniportal approach can also be used successfully in extended lung resections include bronchial sleeve, vascular sleeve, or double sleeve resections [35].

As discussed, the postoperative results of VATS compared to open lobectomy have been confirmed in the various studies. Inexperienced centers, VATS lobectomy is successfully applied not only in the early stage but also in the surgical treatment of locally advanced lung cancer.

7. Conclusions

Minimally invasive surgical approaches have become the preferred choice in many diagnostic and therapeutic surgical interventions in today's thoracic surgery.

However, patient safety should always be prioritized in the selection of the surgical method. Intraoperative complications, especially for major lung resections, carry a high risk of morbidity and mortality. Therefore, it is very important for the surgeon to complete the learning curve in minimally invasive surgery.

It is an indisputable fact that technology directly affects surgical techniques and equipment therefore, as long as technological developments continue, minimally invasive approaches will keep up its evolution.

Conflict of interest

The authors declare no conflict of interest.

Acronyms and abbreviations

CT	Computed tomography
EBUS	Endobronchial ultrasound
EUS	Endoscopic ultrasound
MRI	Magnetic resonance imaging
NSCLC	Non-small cell lung cancer
PET	Positron emission tomography
VATS	Video-assisted thoracic surgery

Author details

Güntuğ Batıhan* and Kenan Can Ceylan
University of Health Sciences Turkey, Dr. Suat Seren Chest Diseases and Chest Surgery Training and Research Center, İzmir, Turkey

*Address all correspondence to: gbatihan@hotmail.com

References

[1] Reddy RV. The advantages of VATS: a systematic review. Thorax 2005;60:238.

[2] Villamizar NR, Darrabie MD, Burfeind WR, et al. Thoracoscopic lobectomy is associated with lower morbidity compared with thoracotomy. J Thorac Cardiovasc Surg 2009;138: 419-25.

[3] Paul S, Altorki NK, Sheng S, et al. Thoracoscopic lobectomy is associated with lower morbidity than open lobectomy: a propensity-matched analysis from the STS database. J Thorac Cardiovasc Surg 2010;139:366-78.

[4] Petersen RP, Pham D, Burfeind WR, et al. Thoracoscopic lobectomy facilitates the delivery of chemotherapy after resection for lung cancer. Ann Thorac Surg 2007;83:1245-9; discussion 1250.

[5] Swanson SJ, Meyers BF, Gunnarsson CL, et al. Video-assisted thoracoscopic lobectomy is less costly and morbid than open lobectomy: a retrospective multiinstitutional database analysis. Ann Thorac Surg 2012;93:1027-32.

[6] Ng CS, Whelan RL, Lacy AM, et al. Is minimal access surgery for cancer associated with immunologic benefits? World J Surg 2005;29:975-81.

[7] Paget S. The surgery of the chest. Bristol, England: John Wright & Co.; 1896.

[8] Kittle CF. The history of lobectomy and segmentectomy including sleeve resection. Chest Surg Clin N Am 2000;10:105-130.

[9] Chang JHAPTSENMaTANYS-VBH, 1991. 25-29. Print.

[10] Whittemore W. The treatment of such cases of chronic suppurative bronchiectasis as are limited to one lobe of the lung. Ann Surg 1927;86:219-226.

[11] Smith A. Development of lung surgery in the United Kingdom. Thorax 1982;37:161-168.

[12] Nissen R. Development of total pneumonectomy. Am J Surg 1949;78:816-820.

[13] Lewis RJ, Caccavale RJ, Sisler GE, et al. One hundred consecutive patients undergoing video-assisted thoracic operations. Ann Thorac Surg 1992;54: 421-426.

[14] McKenna RJ. Lobectomy by video-assisted thoracic surgery with mediastinal node sampling for lung cancer. J Thorac Cardiovasc Surg 1994;107:879-882.

[15] Sihoe AD, Yim AP. Video-assisted pulmonary resections. In: Patterson FG, Cooper JD, Deslauriers J. eds. Thoracic Surgery (3rd Edition). Philadelphia: Elsevier, 2008:970-88.

[16] Sihoe AD. The Evolution of VATS Lobectomy. In: Cardoso P. eds. Topics in Thoracic Surgery. Rijeka: Intech, 2011:181-210.

[17] Rocco G, Khalil M, Jutley R. Uniportal video-assisted thoracoscopic surgery wedge lung biopsy in the diagnosis of interstitial lung diseases. J Thorac Cardiovasc Surg 2005;129: 947-8.

[18] Gonzalez D, Paradela M, Garcia J, et al. Single-port video-assisted thoracoscopic lobectomy. Interact Cardiovasc Thorac Surg 2011;12:514-5.

[19] Gonzalez-Rivas D, Paradela M, Fernandez R, et al. Uniportal video-assisted thoracoscopic lobectomy: two years of experience. Ann Thorac Surg 2013;95:426-32.

[20] Sihoe AD, Hsin MK, Yu PS. Needlescopic video-assisted thoracic surgery pleurodesis for primary pneumothorax. Multimed Man Cardiothorac Surg. 2014 Jun 25;2014:mmu012.

[21] Kim TS, Kim KH, An CH, Kim JS. Single center experiences of needlescopic grasper assisted single incision laparoscopic cholecystectomy for gallbladder benign disease: comparison with conventional 3-port laparoscopic cholecystectomy. Ann Surg Treat Res. 2016;91:233-8.

[22] Inoue S, Kajiwara M, Teishima J, Matsubara A. Needlescopicassisted laparoendoscopic single-site adrenalectomy. Asian J Surg. 2016;39:6-11.

[23] Chen JS, Hsu HH, Kuo SW, Tsai PR, Chen RJ, Lee JM, Lee YC. Needlescopic versus conventional video-assisted thoracic surgery for primary spontaneous pneumothorax: a comparative study. Ann Thorac Surg. 2003 Apr;75(4):1080-5.

[24] Ko HJ, Chiang XH, Yang SM, Yang MC. Needlescopic-assisted thoracoscopic pulmonary anatomical lobectomy and segmentectomy for lung cancer: a bridge between multiportal and uniportal thoracoscopic surgery. Surg Today. 2019 Jan;49(1):49-55.

[25] Augustin F, Bodner J. Robotic-assisted thoracic surgery: a helpful tool or just another expensive gadget? J Thorac Dis 2017;9(9):2881-2883.

[26] Veronesi G. Robotic surgery for the treatment of early-stage lung cancer. Curr Opin Oncol 2013;25:107-14.

[27] Augustin F, Bodner J, Maier H, et al. Robotic-assisted minimally invasive vs. thoracoscopic lung lobectomy: comparison of perioperative results in a learning curve setting. Langenbecks Arch Surg 2013;398:895-901.

[28] Howington JA. The role of VATS for staging and diagnosis in patients with non-small cell lung cancer. Semin Thorac Cardiovasc Surg. 2007 Fall;19(3):212-6. doi: 10.1053/j.semtcvs.2007.07.007.

[29] Simon C. Y. Chow, Calvin S. H. Ng. Recent developments in video-assisted thoracoscopic surgery for pulmonary nodule management. J Thorac Dis 2016;8(Suppl 6):S509-S516

[30] Chang AC, Yee J, Orringer MB, Iannettoni MD. Diagnostic thoracoscopic lung biopsy: an outpatient experience. Ann Thorac Surg. 2002 Dec;74(6):1942-6; discussion 1946-7.

[31] Ciriaco P, Negri G, Puglisi A, Nicoletti R, Del Maschio A, Zannini P. Video-assisted thoracoscopic surgery for pulmonary nodules: rationale for preoperative computed tomography-guided hookwire localization. Eur J Cardiothorac Surg. 2004 Mar;25(3): 429-33.

[32] Lenglinger FX, Schwarz CD, Artmann W. Localization of pulmonary nodules before thoracoscopic surgery: value of percutaneous staining with methylene blue. AJR Am J Roentgenol. 1994 Aug;163(2):297-300.

[33] Martins FK, Oliveira GA, da Silva TK, Bello RM, Coelho JC, Gelatti A, Lewgoy J, Pasa MB. Nodule marking strategies: cost-benefit. J Vis Surg 2018;4:220

[34] Lewis RJ, Caccavale RJ, Bocage JP, Widmann MD. Video-assisted thoracic surgical non-rib spreading simultaneously stapled lobectomy: a more patient-friendly oncologic resection. Chest. 1999 Oct;116(4):1119-24.

[35] Gonzalez-Rivas D, Fieira E, Delgado M, de la Torre M, Mendez L, Fernandez R. Uniportal video-assisted thoracoscopic sleeve lobectomy and other complex resections. J Thorac Dis. 2014;6(Suppl 6):S674-S681.

Chapter 6

Minimally-Invasive Surgery of Mitral Valve. State of the Art

Daniel Pereda and Elena Sandoval

Abstract

Minimally-invasive mitral valve surgery has been in development during the last thirty years and now allows to perform mitral and tricuspid interventions, coronary bypass surgery, repair of congenital heart defects and more. Current state-of-the-art technology and clinical knowledge make possible to offer this approach in expert centers to a growing number of patients, who benefit from its advantages. Minimally-invasive mitral surgery is becoming the best option to repair que mitral valve and patients are able to recover better and faster than after conventional surgery without compromising quality of the repair. With the aid of high-definition 3D visualization and specifically designed instruments, including robotic telemanipulation, thoracoscopic and robotic surgery performed this way require only small incisions in the right chest. In the present chapter we will expose the current state of this field, going into detail regarding patient selection and operative techniques, and also reviewing the requirements for building a successful program.

Keywords: Mitral valve, endoscopic, robotic, minimally-invasive

1. Introduction

Modern minimally-invasive mitral surgery started in the mid 90's with the arrival of technical improvements in peripheral cannulation for cardiopulmonary bypass, vacuum-assisted drainage and specifically-designed long-shafted instruments, that allowed surgeons to safely perform mitral interventions through small anterolateral thoracotomies using thoracoscopic visualization [1].

Another major step forward in this field was the development of endoaortic balloon occlusion devices that, introduced through the femoral artery and positioned in the ascending aorta, allowed to occlude the aorta and to administer antegrade cardioplegia to arrest the heart. The safe and effective utilization of this device required close coordination between the anesthesiologist, the perfusionist and the surgeon, together with continuous monitorization of its correct position by transesophageal echocardiography and avoid its migration during the case, with the risks of injuring the aortic valve (proximal migration) or the occlusion of the head vessels in the aortic arch (distal migration). There were also risks of embolization of atherosclerotic debris and even of aortic dissection, making the selection of adequate candidates for the procedure of paramount importance. Another strategy that evolved to simplify the operation consisted in cross-clamping the aorta using specifically designed transthoracic vascular clamps. These can be rigid or articulated and are introduced either from the working port or using a separate incision in the chest, allowing an external occlusion of the aorta as in conventional surgery. This

IntechOpen

strategy reduces the complexity and costs of the procedure and avoids the risks involved with the use of the endoaortic balloon.

Two more percutaneous tools have been developed to facilitate minimally-invasive operations, both designed to be inserted by the anesthesiologist through the right jugular vein, the "endovent": a suction catheter introduced in the pulmonary artery to reduce the blood return from the pulmonary veins into the left atrium during surgery, and the "endoplegia": a catheter placed inside the coronary sinus to administer retrograde cardioplegia throughout the case.

Further refinements and technological developments included specifically-designed instruments, the introduction of high-definition videothoracoscopy and, more recently, 3D visualization. All these advancements facilitate the performance of this complex procedures and try to mitigate the learning curve involved. Despite these refinements, thoracoscopic mitral repair has not been widely adopted by the cardiac surgery community, and difficult procedures such as complex repairs, reoperations, combined ablation and multivalvular procedures are mostly performed in few, high-volume centers.

Robotic surgery was developed in the late 90's and the first mitral repair and mitral replacement with the da Vinci system (Intuitive Surgical. CA, USA) were performed in Europe by Carpentier [2] and Mohr [3] in 1998 and in the USA by Chitwood [4] in 2000, respectively.

Robotic mitral surgery has slowly expanded worldwide and it is currently the preferred surgical approach for mitral repair in many programs. The only robotic platform in clinical use for cardiac surgery is the DaVinci system (Intuitive Surgical. CA, USA), which is currently in its 4th generation with the X and the Xi systems. These two systems are capable to perform cardiac surgery and provide some advantages with respect to previous models. However, many groups still rely on the previous generation, the Si, which is particularly useful for coronary revascularization since it has dedicated instruments such as the coronary endo-stabilizer, that are not provided for the newest generation.

Robotic technology allows the surgeon to regain much of the dexterity lost by the use of long-shafted instruments and provides superb high-definition 3D visualization with up to 10x magnification. This technology provides unparalleled precision inside the chest and a range of movement even wider than that of the human hand [5]. Another great advantage of robotic telemanipulation in the field of mitral surgery comes with the use of a third robotic arm equipped with the dynamic atrial retractor. This instrument provides outstanding exposure of the valve that adapts to every patient's particular anatomy and is controlled with the same precision and dexterity as the rest of surgical instruments. As exposure and visualization of the valve and subvalvular apparatus is better, all repair techniques can be robotically performed, including the most complex ones such as papillary muscle repositioning or the sliding leaflet plasty. Reported results in experienced centers show excellent results, both in repair rate and postoperative complications. Robotic mitral surgery has demonstrated shorter intensive care unit (ICU) and hospital length of stay, better quality of life postoperatively and better cosmesis, as compared to conventional surgery [6, 7].

In this chapter, we will review in detail all the key points of current state-of-the-art minimally invasive mitral surgery, both thoracoscopic and robotic, from the indications and the evaluation of candidates to a step-by-step walkthrough of both techniques.

2. Preoperative evaluation

All patients should undergo a high-quality comprehensive transthoracic or transesophageal echocardiographic evaluation to have a good understanding of their particular valve disease before the operation. Echocardiography also provides valuable clues to avoid technique-related complications such as systolic anterior motion (SAM) and helps in the selection of the most adequate type and size of annuloplasty prosthesis.

Proper patient selection is crucial to avoid postoperative complications. Minimally-invasive surgery is more difficult in morbidly obese patients and in those with small thoracic cavities. Other anatomical issues that affect port placement or may limit the movements of the robotic arms include: scoliosis, pectus excavatum, phrenic nerve palsy and intrathoracic herniation of abdominal viscera. History of prior thoracic surgery, radiation or thoracic trauma should be ruled out preoperatively and may contraindicate a thoracoscopic or robotic surgery [8–10].

The need for peripheral cannulation for cardiopulmonary bypass mandates a thorough evaluation of the vascular system and an adequate size of the femoral vessels. A detailed physical examination and preoperative thoracic, abdominal and pelvic computed tomography angiograms are essential to ensure a safe operation. Evaluation of the venous system for signs of thrombosis or occlusion (interrupted inferior vena cava, presence of cava filters or extrinsic compression) is also achieved with these examinations. Patients with cardiovascular risk factors should undergo a preoperative coronary angiogram (with coronary catheterization or computed tomography angiography) to rule out ischemic heart disease.

Minimally-invasive surgery requires single-lung ventilation at different moments during the operation. Single-lung ventilation causes hypoxia and hypercarbia and increased pulmonary artery pressure. Patients with chronic pulmonary disease or pulmonary hypertension should undergo further testing to determine if they can tolerate this safely. Single-lung ventilation can be reduced or even avoided at the expense of longer cardiopulmonary bypass duration, so a tailored risk–benefit evaluation should be performed for these patients [11].

2.1 Indications and contraindications

Minimally-invasive mitral surgery follows the same indications that apply to conventional surgery, as described in the current guidelines published by the major European and American scientific societies of cardiac surgery and cardiology [12, 13].

Minimally-invasive surgery has some contraindications, detailed below [8–10]:

- Coronary artery disease requiring revascularization.
- Severe peripheral vascular disease or aneurysms of the descending thoracic or abdominal aorta.
- Prior right chest surgery.
- Severe chest wall deformities.
- Ascending aorta dilatation >45 mm or calcification.
- Moderate to severe aortic stenosis or regurgitation.
- Severe calcification of the mitral annulus.
- Severe pulmonary dysfunction or pulmonary hypertension.

All the prior situations described would difficult basic steps for a minimally invasive surgery and deem the operation unsafe. However, certain aspects of the technique, such as peripheral cannulation or cardioplegia administration, can be modified in order to adapt to some of these situations and still be able to offer a minimally invasive approach.

3. Fundamentals of minimally-invasive mitral surgery

Both thoracoscopic and robotic approaches to repair the mitral valve share a basic common set of techniques, skills, tools, anesthetic management and mitral repair techniques. These include the use of retrograde peripheral perfusion, similar options for myocardial protection, working with thoracic ports, thoracoscopic visualization instead of direct vision, and the use of specifically designed surgical instruments.

In addition to these intraoperative and more technical aspects, both approaches also share a similar philosophy in terms of patient selection and postoperative management to assure a successful outcome and an improved postoperative recovery, with a faster return to normal activities after surgery.

3.1 Mitral repair techniques used in minimally-invasive surgery

We follow the same basic principles of mitral repair regardless of the approach used, conventional or minimally-invasive, as established by Carpentier over 30 years ago [14]. This can be summarized in these principles:

1. Preservation or restoration of normal leaflet mobility.

2. Creation of a good coaptation between the anterior and the posterior leaflet along the entire coaptation line.

3. Remodeling and stabilization of the mitral annulus using an annuloplasty band or ring.

To achieve a successful mitral repair program, it is mandatory to clearly understand both the vast array of mitral pathology and to master a large armamentarium of techniques to address every specific case. A comprehensive understanding of mitral pathology is imperative to follow a structured analysis, as proposed by Carpentier, clearly distinguishing between etiology, lesions and dysfunctions. Etiology is the cause of the valvular problem (e.g., fibroelastic deficiency, infective endocarditis, ischemic heart disease), lesions are the results of the disease (e.g., chordal rupture, leaflet perforation, annular calcification) and the dysfunction is the result of the lesions (e.g., leaflet prolapse, restricted leaflet closure) (**Figure 1**). This may appear simple, but it is not uncommon to see these three concepts mixed up when evaluating echocardiography reports, discussing with other surgeons and cardiology colleagues and reading the medical literature. Following this approach to mitral disease, we are able to follow a systematic methodology to describe the problem and solve it.

Most of the techniques described and used in open surgery to repair the mitral valve can also be used successfully in minimally-invasive surgery, both thoracoscopic and robotic, but some adaptations must be implemented to facilitate its use in these approaches.

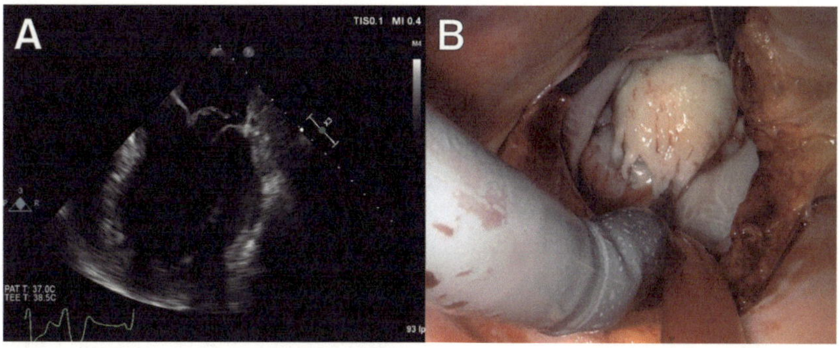

Figure 1.
A shows a two-chamber view of the preoperative transesophageal echocardiography where a flail anterior leaflet due to chordal rupture can be seen. B shows an intraoperative view of the anterior mitral leaflet of the same patient during robotic mitral repair, confirming the preoperative echocardiographic findings.

3.1.1 Triangular and quadrangular resections

Triangular resections are ideal to treat a localized prolapse of the posterior leaflet, when the prolapsing segment involves only one scallop without affecting the complete length of its free edge. This technique is very well suited for thoracoscopic and robotic surgery. The resection is triangular in shape with its base at the free edge and extending towards the annulus up to 2/3 to 3/4 of the leaflet height. Ideally, the edges of the resection should be convex towards each other and care must be taken not to resect too much of the free edge, to avoid producing a "curtain effect" upon re-approximation. Reconstruction of the leaflet can be accomplished with interrupted or running sutures. If the latter is preferred, the surgeon must avoid a purse-string effect that could impair leaflet mobility. We prefer to use a double running technique using 4/0 polypropylene sutures. Some surgeons prefer using 5/0 sutures, but we only use them when the leaflets are very thin (**Figure 2**).

Quadrangular resections are preferred when large portions of the posterior leaflet are prolapsing with great excess of tissue. In this technique the resection is extended all the way to the posterior annulus in a rectangular or trapezoidal shape. In order to avoid excessive tension upon reapproximation, the posterior annulus is plicated using interrupted, pledgeted 2/0 braided sutures. This maneuver excludes a portion of the dilated annulus from the final repaired valve, increasing the amount of annular remodeling. In complex cases, where a very large portion of the posterior must be resected, the "sliding plasty" technique allows reconstruction without the need for excessive annular plication. In this technique the base of posterior leaflet on both ends of the resection are detached from the annulus and advanced centrally during reattachment.

3.1.2 Chordal replacement

Neochordal implantation using polytetrafluoroethylene (PTFE) sutures has gained great popularity in the treatment of mitral prolapse, particularly on the anterior leaflet. There are some reasons for the enthusiastic adoption of this technique, particularly in minimally-invasive approaches:

- Simplicity: is a simple way to treat complex problems.

- Availability: neochords can be easily constructed in any number and length to accommodate any particular anatomy.

- Reversibility: in case of a suboptimal result, it is easy to remove the neochord and replace it with another at any moment during the operation. In contrast, once a resection is performed, this cannot be undone.

- Precision: adjusting the length of the chords allows the optimization of coaptation, this can be performed during water test to simulate systolic closure. In cases of very redundant leaflets, applying more restriction on the posterior leaflet by shortening the neochords can prevent SAM.

- Reproducibility and good long-term durability: using a standardized technique, mitral repair with this approach has proven extremely effective and durable.

Neochords are constructed using 4/0 PTFE sutures that are anchored in the tip of the papillary muscle and the free edge of the prolapsing leaflet (**Figure 2**). Our technique of choice consists in passing both ends of the suture with a PTFE pledget through the tip of the target papillary muscle head. We do not tie the suture down in the papillary muscle to allow both ends of the suture to automatically adjust their length, so that tension is equally distributed among them. Then, both chords are passed twice around the free edge of the prolapsing segment in a "figure-of-eight" fashion and chordal length is adjusted visually, taking into account the distance to annular plane, the length of the normal chords on both sides of the prolapsing segment and the excess of leaflet tissue. The valve is then tested using saline to fill the ventricle and the final length adjustments are made to optimize the depth of

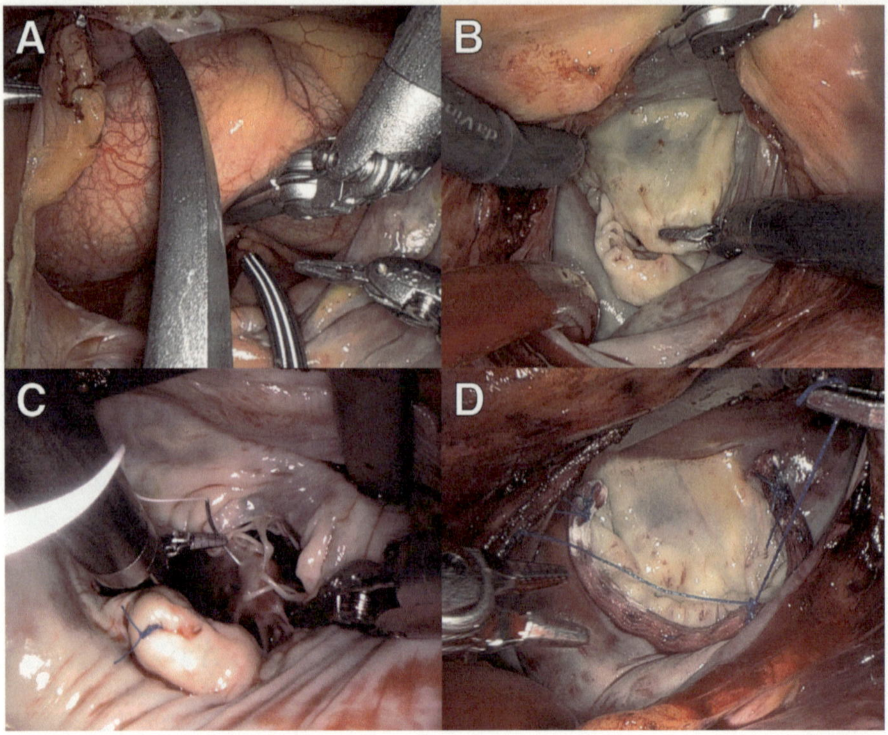

Figure 2.
Displays different steps of a minimally-invasive mitral repair: A shows the placement of the transthoracic aortic clamp in the ascending aorta through the transverse sinus with the aid of three robotic arms. B represents the initial surgical valve analysis, showing a posterior leaflet prolapse of its central scallop. C shows the surgical exposition of the posteromedial papillary muscle during the implantation of a PTFE neochord. D shows the final aspect of a repaired valve after the annuloplasty has been performed using a flexible band implanted using continuous sutures.

coaptation and the position of the closure line. Once the desired result is achieved, the chords are tied on the atrial side of the leaflet to secure the resulting length.

3.1.3 Mitral annuloplasty

As discussed earlier, we implant an annuloplasty ring in nearly all repairs. The choice of the ring depends on the etiology and the disfunction of the patient. We favor flexible bands for cases with mitral prolapse and complete rigid rings for functional regurgitation and whenever significant leaflet tethering is present. Sizing of the ring follows a standardized method, taking into account the intertrigonal distance and most importantly, the surface area of the anterior leaflet. A small under or oversizing from this initial measurement can be added to accommodate the repair according to some particular features of the case such as the perceived risk of SAM, very significant excess of tissue on the leaflets and leaflet tethering due to ventricular dilatation.

Annuloplasty rings can be implanted using interrupted or running sutures. For complete rings and bands implanted thoracoscopically or through median sternotomy, we favor the interrupted suturing technique using 2–0 braided sutures. On robotic cases, we prefer to use the running suturing technique with monofilament sutures (barbed polybutester or PTFE) instead, due to the significant gain in time and the simplicity it provides while working with the bedside surgeon during the implant. This running suturing technique is facilitated by the greater dexterity of the robotic system and the main drawback is that it may be more difficult to judge the distribution of sutures along the annulus and the band, particularly in cases with very dilated annulus requiring significant annular remodeling (**Figure 2**).

4. Operative technique

4.1 Common steps for robotic and thoracoscopic surgery: patient preparation and cardiopulmonary bypass

After induction of anesthesia, the patient is intubated and a transesophageal echocardiography (TEE) probe is positioned. Intubation can be performed either with a double-lumen endotracheal tube or with a single lumen tube and a bronchial occluder with a balloon. The patient is positioned in supine, as close as possible to the right side of the surgical table, the right chest is slightly elevated placing a blanket roll along the right hemithorax and the right arm is allowed to fall below the right chest to expose the lateral chest and the axilla. Care must be taken to protect the arm to avoid neural injuries due to compression against the structure of the table.

Cardiopulmonary bypass (CPB) is commonly instituted with cannulation of the right common femoral vessels, using a small 3 cm incision to expose both vessels (**Figure 3**). Dissection is kept to a minimum to avoid damage to the surrounding neural structures and to decrease the risk of seroma formation after surgery. Only the anterior wall of the vessels is exposed, and two 5/0 polypropylene purse-strings are placed in a rectangular fashion following the long axis of both vessels. After heparinization, the femoral vein is cannulated using the Seldinger technique and a guidewire is advanced under TEE guidance into the superior vena cava. Then the puncture site is sequentially enlarged using dilators and finally a 25F multiperforated venous cannula is, under TEE guidance, introduced and placed with its tips 3 to 5 cm inside the superior vena cava (SVC). After securing the

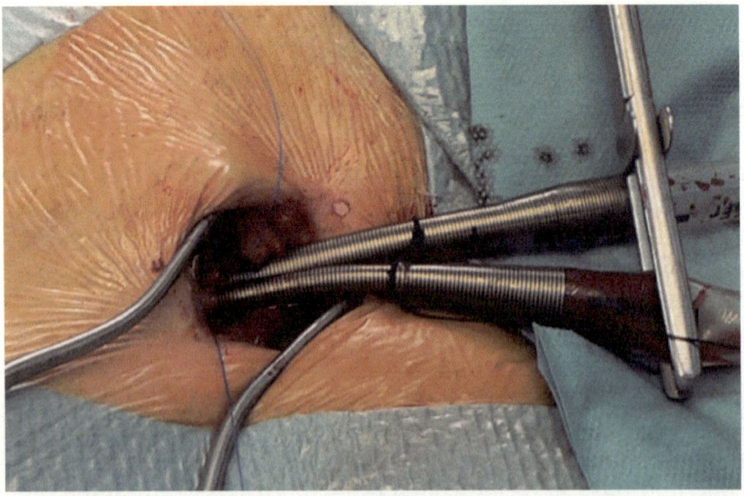

Figure 3.
Shows the right common femoral artery and vein cannulated for cardiopulmonary bypass.

venous cannula to the skin with stay sutures, arterial cannulation is performed following the same technique described, using TEE to verify the position of the guidewire in the descending aorta. The diameter of the vessel is the sole determinant of the size chosen for the arterial cannula and typically ranges from 15F to 19F. We never oversize the arterial cannula and prefer to use a 6-8 mm Dacron side-graft if in doubt. In rare cases when we have to use a cannula that completely occludes the lumen (as in obese patients with poor femoral arteries) and the planned procedure is long, we place a distal perfusion line to prevent limb ischemia and a postoperative compartment syndrome. For this purpose, we use a 6F introducer connected to the arterial line through a side port.

Using this technique, we do not need routine cannulation of the jugular vein for mitral surgery, but it is crucial to always use vacuum-assisted drainage in the venous line and to make sure the venous cannula is correctly positioned inside the superior vena cava to avoid its occlusion by the Chitwood clamp when the atrial retractor is placed in the left atrium and pulled anteriorly to expose the valve.

4.2 Endoscopic surgery

4.2.1 Port placement and initial steps

Under left-lung ventilation the working port is created in the 4th intercostal space performing a 3-4 cm incision around the level of the anterior axillary line and a soft-tissue retractor (Alexis XSl, Applied Medical, CA) is placed to prevent inadvertently introducing fatty tissue or debris in the cardiac chambers during the introduction of surgical instruments, sutures or valvular prostheses. Then, a 5 mm trocar is placed in the third intercostal space along the anterior axillary line and CO2 is continuously insufflated (4 L/min) throughout the entire operation, to create an intrathoracic CO2 environment that reduces the risk of air embolism after releasing the aortic clamp. This trocar is used to introduce a 5 mm 30-degree videothoracoscopic HD camera to guide the procedure and the camera is held by an articulated arm placed in the right side of the head piece of the surgical table (**Figure 4**). An 11 mm trocar is placed in the 6th intercostal space, mid-axillary line. We use this second trocar to exteriorize retraction sutures (placed in the diaphragm and in the lower portion of the pericardium) and to introduce the left atrial vent line. After the

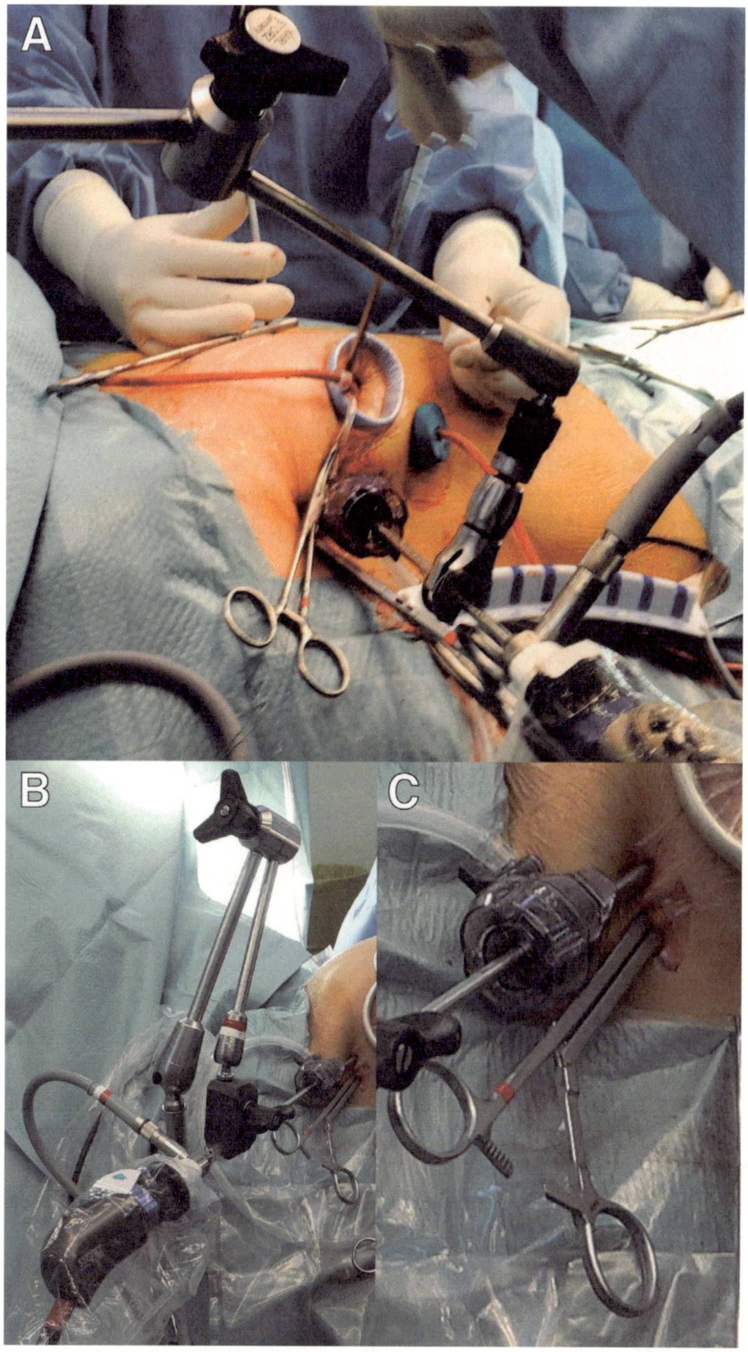

Figure 4.
Presents the final set-up of an endoscopic surgery. A shows the surgical field with all the ports during a mitral repair through a periareolar incision. In this image the surgeon is using two long-shafted instruments through the working port and the assistant is moving the left atrial retractor to improve exposure. B shows the thoracoscopic camera held in position by an articulated arm. C show how the transthoracic clamp is inserted below the camera trocar.

procedure is completed, a 28F chest tube will be passed through this trocar and left in the pleural space. If diaphragmatic retraction is needed (>75% of cases), a pledgeted “2/0” PTFE suture is placed and tied in the central tendon, taking great care not to damage the liver during this maneuver. The traction suture is exteriorized through the 11 mm trocar and tension is applied to improve exposure. Then, the pericardium completely opened in its lateral aspect with a longitudinal incision performed at least 3 cm anterior to the phrenic nerve. Two PTFE stay sutures are placed near the cranial and caudal ends of the posterior edge of the pericardium and exteriorized using the 11 mm trocar for the caudal suture and a transthoracic puncture just cranial and posterior to the working port, in the mid axillary line.

After opening the pericardium and placing the stay sutures in the diaphragm and the pericardium, the aortic cross-clamp is inserted through a 5mmm incision in the 3rd intercostal space mid-axillary line (**Figure 4**). A curved Chitwood clamp is advanced inside the pericardium and placed across the ascending aorta, with its lower jaw placed inside the transverse sinus under thoracoscopic vision and using blunt instruments (typically a thoracoscopic suction cannula) to push the aorta anteriorly. Once the aortic clamp is in place, a pledgeted purse string is placed in the ascending aorta and a long cardioplegic needle is inserted through the working port under thoracoscopic vision. At this point, cardiopulmonary bypass is initiated and, upon reaching full systemic flow, the ventilator is disconnected and the aorta is cross-clamped.

Our technique for myocardial protection consists on antegrade administration of cold blood cardioplegia (Buckberg's technique) after cross-clamping the aorta and repeated every 20 minutes thereafter. During cardioplegia infusion, the left atrium is opened just below the interatrial septum and the left atrial vent is introduced and placed in the left pulmonary veins to maintain a bloodless surgical field. The size of the left atrial retractor blade is selected at this moment and the stem of the retractor is placed under thoracoscopic control, typically through the 5th intercostal space along the midclavicular line. The retractor is then assembled inside the thorax and placed inside the left atrium. Retraction is then applied to achieve an adequate exposure of the mitral valve. The atrial retractor is held in place using a second articulated arm placed on the left side or the table.

4.2.2 Completion of the operation

After achieving the mitral repair or replacement, the left atriotomy is closed. Our preference for this is to use monofilament sutures (barbed polybutester or PTFE) using two sutures secured at both ends of the atriotomy and sutured towards the center. While finishing this step, the left atrial vent line is removed so blood is allowed to start filling the left cardiac chambers to begin de-airing. After closing the atriotomy, suction is applied in the root vent line and both lungs are manually inflated to remove as much air as possible from the heart and pulmonary veins before releasing the aortic cross-clamp. To further assist this process, the venous line can be intermittently clamped to allow blood to fill the right heart and the lungs and push air out from the heart. After completing de-airing, the aortic clamp is released and the heart is reperfused. We do not put pacing wires routinely after isolated mitral mitral repair in patients without previous rhythm abnormalities; if they are required, they can be placed in the right atrial wall and/or on the right ventricular wall. After normal rhythm is restored, and preliminary echocardiographic evaluation of valvular and ventricular function is satisfactory, the patient is weaned from cardiopulmonary bypass in the usual fashion. Our preference is to remove the aortic root vent after echocardiographic evaluation of the result is completed under a short period of full-flow cardiopulmonary bypass, to facilitate the removal of the cannula and the repair of the entry site with low aortic pressure and reduced pulsatility. After this is completed satisfactorily, the patient is weaned from cardiopulmonary bypass and decannulated, and protamine is given. All ports are removed under thoracoscopic control to avoid any port site bleeding, and pericardial (19F Blake drain) and pleural (28F curved chest tube) draining tubes are implanted using the port incisions. The pericardium is loosely approximated with two or three interrupted sutures to avoid the low risk of cardiac herniation and facilitate reoperation, should future procedures be needed.

After cannulas are removed from the femoral vessels, the purse strings are tied and both cannulation sites are reinforced with 5/0 polypropylene sutures. After hemostasis is accomplished all incisions are closed in the usual fashion and the patient is usually extubated in the operating room immediately after the operation is completed.

4.3 Robotic surgery

Most of the preparations and initial steps of the operation are the same as described before in detail for the endoscopic surgical procedure. In short, the patient is positioned in supine with mild right chest elevation, on demand single-lung mechanical ventilation is prepared and cardiopulmonary bypass is established using the right femoral vessels.

The placement of the trocars for the robotic arms starts with the introduction of an 8 mm trocar in the 4th intercostal space between the mid clavicular and the anterior axillary lines using blunt dissection; this will serve as the camera port. After insertion, the camera port is connected to a CO_2 line to create a controlled pneumothorax using a pressure limit of 7-10 mmHg. The scope is inserted in the trocar and the right pleural space inspected for adhesions. Under thoracoscopic visualization, 3 angiocaths are inserted at the 4th, 6th and 7th intercostal spaces in the posterior axillary line; these will be used to exteriorize the traction sutures placed on the diaphragm and the pericardium. It is important to keep these catheters occluded to avoid losing CO_2 during this phase. Then, the right arm trocar is inserted in the 6th intercostal space, approximately 2 cm posterior to the camera port. Thereafter, the left arm trocar in inserted in the 2nd or 3rd intercostal space at the same level as the

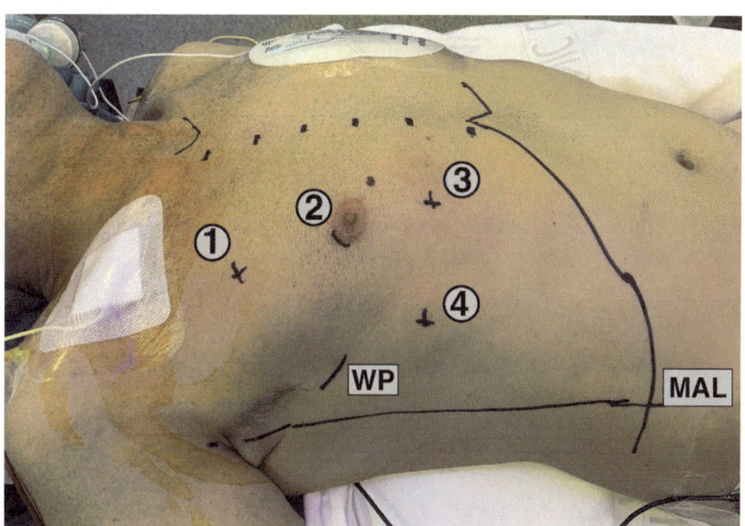

Figure 5.
This picture shows a patient set-up for a robotic mitral repair. Markings in the chest reveal the surgical landmarks used for port placement and the anticipated location of the four arms of the robot. The location of the working port (WP) is also shown, and the mid-axillary line (MAL) is drawn to help in the placement of the retraction sutures for the diaphragm and the pericardium.

camera port. Finally, the trocar for the atrial retractor is inserted in the 6th intercostal space just medial to the mid clavicular line, avoiding injuring the internal thoracic artery. All trocars are inserted under direct vision using the scope. Once all trocars are in place, a 2-3 cm thoracotomy is performed around 3 cm lateral to the camera port, in the same intercostal space, to serve as the working port. After achieving proper hemostasis, a soft tissue retractor is applied leaving a suction catheter outside, that will be used as a left atrial vent during the operation (**Figure 5**).

Once all thoracic steps are completed, heparin can be administered and the femoral vessels are cannulated as described earlier in detail. Once both cannulas are secured and connected to the CPB circuit, the DaVinci system can be docked to the patient. It is extremely important to connect the trocars in the direction they will move to avoid potential conflicts between the robotic arms. The camera port is connected to arm number 2 and, under endoscopic visualization, instruments are placed in arms 1 and 4 and introduced inside the thorax for the console surgeon control (**Figure 6**). At this stage CPB can be started, although in some patients with

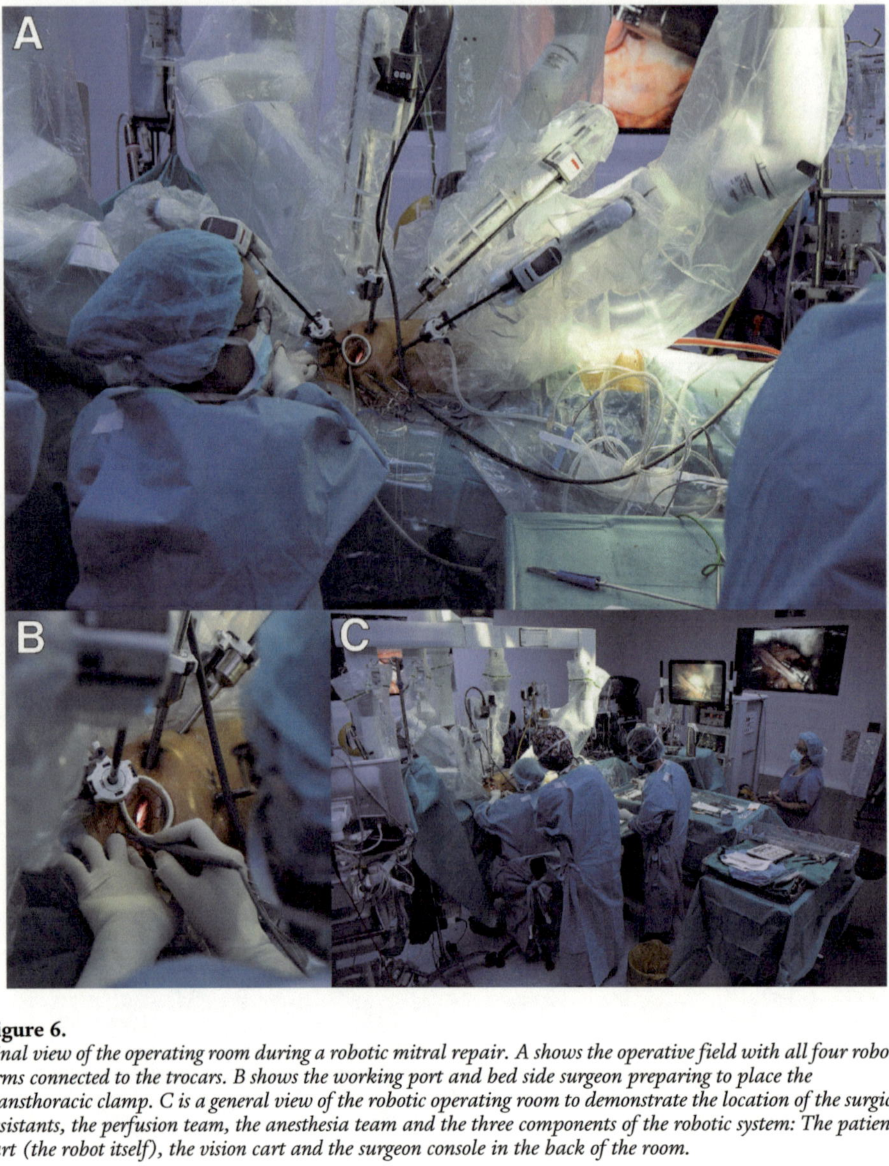

Figure 6.
Final view of the operating room during a robotic mitral repair. A shows the operative field with all four robotic arms connected to the trocars. B shows the working port and bed side surgeon preparing to place the transthoracic clamp. C is a general view of the robotic operating room to demonstrate the location of the surgical assistants, the perfusion team, the anesthesia team and the three components of the robotic system: The patient cart (the robot itself), the vision cart and the surgeon console in the back of the room.

excellent anatomy the pericardium can be opened and the diaphragm retracted before starting CPB. For diaphragmatic and pericardial retraction, we normally use a 2/0 PTFE sutures as described in the thoracoscopic procedure. These sutures exit the chest through the angiocaths placed at the beginning of the operation.

The atrial retractor is inserted under direct vision on the robotic arm number 3, and used to separate the aorta from the SVC to expose the transverse sinus. Placement of the transthoracic aortic clamp and cardioplegia administration are performed as described for the endoscopic procedure. The left atrium is incised to expose the mitral valve using the dynamic left atrial retractor (**Figure 2**).

Once the mitral repair or replacement is completed, the left atrium is closed using two running sutures from both ends of the incision as described for the endoscopic procedure. After proper deairing the cross-clamp is removed and the patient is weaned from CPB as described earlier. At this point, the 3rd arm is removed and the trocar is used to insert a 19F Blake drainage inside the pericardium, which is approximated with two sutures. The remaining trocars are removed and checked for bleeding using the camera, and a 24F curved chest tube is inserted in the pleural space using the right arm trocar incision.

5. Results

The primary goal of minimally-invasive mitral repair is, as in open surgery, to achieve a successful and durable valve repair. Despite its perceived technical complexity, experienced centers have reported excellent repair results with 95% freedom from mitral regurgitation at 5 years, even in complex mitral pathology [15–18].

In addition to a durable result, minimally-invasive mitral surgery aims for a faster recovery and higher patient satisfaction as incisions are smaller. Recent series reported higher quality of life and earlier return to work in minimally invasive surgery [16]. Furthermore, several publications have shown that despite longer CPB and aortic-clamp times, minimally invasive surgery is associated with a very low complication rate, reduced blood loss and shorter ICU and in-hospital length of stay [17, 19].

6. Starting a new program

The most successful centers in minimally-invasive mitral surgery are usually high-volume referral centers with vast experience in mitral repair when they started their programs. Minimally invasive surgery, and even more robotic surgery, require developing new skills such as peripheral cannulation, intra-aortic occlusion and the use of thoracoscopic vision and long-shafted instruments. It is not only the surgeon, but the whole operating team (anesthesiologists, perfusionists, Operating room nurses, etc.) that has to learn to use new tools and adapt to new surgical techniques [20].

Based on our own experience, there is an increase in complexity for the whole team when transitioning from open to thoracoscopic surgery, which is even steeper when going further from there to robotic surgery. For this reason, we consider that it is mandatory for the whole surgical team to undergo specific in-depth training in thoracoscopic and robotic cardiac surgery as basic first-step before starting a successful program, either endoscopic or robotic. Training must include the acquisition of the required theoretical knowledge and the progressive achievement of the technical skills required. For the latter, the first step is practicing on simulators and dry lab training. After this step is accomplished, the team can move to higher fidelity wet labs, and training in live, large animal and/or human cadaveric models.

After this basic training the members of the surgical team should do repeated case observation work in experienced large volume institutions and during the first phases of their experience have the aid of expert proctors that can provide the required support to ensure safety for the patient and a profitable learning experience to the team [21].

The best way to stablish a successful program is to avoid overlapping learning curves. Results are better during the initial phases if a robotic program is started by teams with wide experience in mitral repair and there is a strict patient selection protocol. As programs grow in experience, there is a tendency to extend the indication to more complex patients. Surgeons should pay close attention to their results in order to detect any changes on the appearance of complications while extending their inclusion criteria and adjust them accordingly [22, 23].

7. Latest developments and percutaneous devices

Following the expansion of transcatheter devices to treat aortic stenosis, several developments have appeared to repair or replace the mitral valve. The most extended one in the repair group is the MitraClip (Abbott Laboratories. IL, USA), which resembles an edge-to-edge repair. It requires venous access and a transeptal puncture. To date, more than 100000 implants have been performed, mostly on selected patients with secondary mitral regurgitation [24]. More recently, another device using the same concept has been introduced, the Pascal repair system (Edwards Lifesciences. CA, USA) [25].

New transapical devices are trying to resemble mitral repair using neochords, sucha as the Harpoon (Edwards Lifesciences. CA, USA) [26] and the Neochord (Neochord INC. MN, USA) [27] devices, which allow the transpical insertion of neochords on the beating heart under TEE guidance. Both of them require a left mini-thoracotomy and can be used without CPB.

The Cardioband (Edwards Lifesciences. CA, USA) percutaneously delivers an annuloplasty band using a transseptal access. It is anchored with several screws into the mitral annulus and then cinches the valve under TEE guidance.

In the field of percutaneous mitral replacement, the Tendyne bioprosthetic mitral valve system (Abbott Medical Inc. IL, USA) accumulates the larger clinical experience. It is a fully retrievable and repositionable device that is implanted using an off-pump transapical approach.

These and other developments [28, 29] will undoubtedly continue in the future and will reshape the landscape of options to treat the mitral valve for the benefit of patients.

Conflict of interests

The authors declare no conflict of interests.

Author details

Daniel Pereda* and Elena Sandoval
Cardiovascular Surgery Department, Cardiovascular Institute, Hospital Clínic – University of Barcelona, Barcelona, Spain

*Address all correspondence to: dpereda@clinic.cat

References

[1] Fann JI, Pompili MF, Burdon TA, Stevens JH, St Goar FG, Reitz BA. Minimally invasive mitral valve surgery. Semin Thorac Cardiovasc Surg 1997;9: 320-30. PMID: 9352947

[2] Carpentier A, Loulmet D, Aupècle B, Kieffer JP, Tournay D, Guibourt P et al. Computer assisted open heart surgery. First case operated on with success. C R Acad Sci III 1998;321:437-42. doi: 10.1016/s0764-4469(98)80309-0

[3] Mohr FW, Falk V, Diegeler A, et al. Computer-enhanced coronary artery bypass surgery. J Thorac Cardiovasc Surg 1999; 117:1212-4 PMID: 10343274

[4] Chitwood WR, Jr, Nifong LW, Elbeery JE, et al. Robotic mitral valve repair: trapezoidal resection and prosthetic annuloplasty with the da vinci surgical system. J Thorac Cardiovasc Surg 2000; 120:1171-2 doi: 10.1067/mtc.2000.110177.

[5] Gillinov AM, Mihaljevic T, Javadikassari H, Suri RM, Mick SK, Navi JL et al. Early results of robotically assisted mitral valve surgery: Analysis of the first 1000 cases. J Thorac Cardiovasc 2018: 155 (1) 82-91 e2. doi: 10.1016/j.jtcvs.2017.07.037

[6] Suri RM, Antiel RM, Burkhart HM, Huebner M, Li Z, Eton DT et al. Quality of life after early mitral valve repair using conventional and robotic approaches. Ann Thorac Surg 2012: 93: 761-9. doi: 10.1016/j.athoracsur.2011.11.062.

[7] Mihaljevic T, Koprivanac M, Kelava M, Goodman A, Jarrett C, Williams SJ et al. Value of robotically assisted surgery for mitral valve disease. JAMA Surg 2014;149(7):679–86. doi: 10.1001/jamasurg.2013.5680.

[8] Mihaljevic T, Jarrett CM, Gillinov AM, Williams SJ, DeVilliers PA, Stewart WJ, Svensson LG, Sabik JF 3rd, Blackstone EH. Robotic repair of posterior mitral valve prolapse versus conventional approaches: potential realized. *J Thorac Cardiovasc Surg*. 2011;141:72–80. doi: 10.1016/j.jtcvs.2010.09.008.

[9] SSuri RM, Burkhart HM. Optimizing outcomes of robotic mitral valve repair for all prolapse anatomy: the Suri-Burkhart technique. *Ann Cardiothorac Surg*. 2013;2:841–845. doi: 10.3978/j.issn.2225-319X.2013.10.05.

[10] Ailawadi G, Agnihotri AK, Mehall JR, Wolfe JA, Hummel BW, Fayers TM, et al. Minimally invasive mitral valve surgery I: patient selection, evaluation, and planning. Innovations. 2016;11: 243–250. doi: 10.1097/IMI.0000000000000301.

[11] Vernick W, Atluri P. Robotic and minimally invasive cardiac surgery. Anesthesiology Clin 2013 31 299-320. doi: 10.1016/j.anclin.2012.12.002.

[12] Baumgartner H, Falk V, Bax JJ, De Bonis M, Hamm C, Holm PJ et al. 2017 ESC/EACTS Guidelines for the management of valvular heart disease. Eur Heart J 2017; 38: 2739-2791. doi: 10.1093/eurheartj/ehx391.

[13] Otto CM, Nishimura RA, Bonow RO, Carabello BA, Erwin III JP, Gentile F et al. 2020 ACC/AHA Guideline for the management of patients with valvular heart disease. J Am Coll Cardiol. 2021 Feb 2;77(4):e25-e197. doi: 10.1016/j.jacc.2020.11.018

[14] Carpentier A: Cardiac valve surgery: 'The French correction'. *J Thorac Cardiovasc Surg* 1983; **86**: 323- 337. PMID: 6887954

[15] Perier P, Hohenberger W, Lakew F, Batz G, Diegler A. Rate of repair in minimally invasive mitral valve surgery. Ann Cardiothorac Surg 2013: 2 (6): 751-757. doi: 10.3978/j.issn.2225-319X.2013.10.12.

[16] Seeburger J, Borger MA, Falk V, Kuntze T, Czesla M, Walther T et al. Minimally invasive mitral valve repair for mitral regurgitation: results of 1339 consecutive patients. Eur J Cardiothorac Surg 2008 Oct 34(4): 760-5. doi: 10.1016/j.ejcts.2008.05.015.

[17] Suri RM, Taggarse A, Burkhart HM, Daly RC, Mauermann W, Nishimura RA et al. Robotic mitral valve repair for simple and complex degenerative disease. Midterm clinical and echocardiographic quality outcomes. Circulation 2015; 132: 1961-1968. doi: 10.1161/CIRCULATIONAHA.115.017792.

[18] Taui T, Ishikawa N, Horikawa T, Seguchi R, Shigematsu S, Kiuchi R et al. First Major Clinical Outcomes of totally endoscopic robotic mitral valve5 repair in Japan. Circ J 2019; 83: 1668-1673. doi: 10.1253/circj.CJ-19-0284.

[19] Ascaso M, Sandoval E, Quintana E, Vidal B, Castella M, Pereda D. Early and mid-term outcomes of mitral repair due to leaflet prolapse in a national referral center. Rev Esp Cardiol (Engl Ed) 2020; Nov 4: S1885-5857. doi: 10.1016/j.rec.2020.10.002.

[20] Lehr EJ, Guy TS, Smith RL, Grossi EA, Shemin RJ, Rodriguez E, et at. Minimally Invasive Mitral Valve Surgery III. Training and Robotic-Assisted Approaches. Innovations 2016;11: 260–267 doi: 10.1097/IMI.0000000000000299.

[21] Rodriguez E, Nifong LW, Bonatti J, Casula R, Falk V Folliguet TA, et al. Pathway for surgeons and programs to establish and maintain a successful robot-assisted adult cardiac surgery program J Thorac Cardiovasc Surg 2016;152:9-13 doi: 10.1016/j.athoracsur.2016.02.085.

[22] Goodman A, Koprivanac M, Kelava M, Mick SL, Gillinov AM, Rajeswaran J et al. Robotic mitral valve repair. The learning curve. Innovation 2017; 12: 390-7 doi: 10.1097/IMI.0000000000000438.

[23] Kesävuori R, Raivio P, Jokinen JJ, Sahlman A, Teittinen K, Vento A. Early experience with robotic mitral valve repair with intra-aortic occlusion. J Thorac Cardiovasc Surg 2018; 155: 1463-71. doi: 10.1016/j.jtcvs.2017.10.076.

[24] Stone GW, Lindenfeld J, Abraham WT, Kar S, Lim S, Mishell JM et al. Transcatheter mitral-valve repair in patients with heart failure. N Engl J Med 2018; 379: 2307-2318. doi: 10.1056/NEJMoa1806640.

[25] Lim DS, Kar S, Spargias K, et al. Transcatheter valve repair for patients with mitral regurgitation: 30-day results of the CLASP study. JACC Cardiovasc Interv. 2019;12(14): 1369-1378 doi: 10.1016/j.jcin.2019.04.034.

[26] Gammie JS, Wilson P, Bartus K, Gackowski A, Hung J, D'Ambra MV, et al. Transapical beating-heart mitral vavle repair with an expanded polytetrafluoroëthylene cordal implantation device. Circulation 2016; 134: 189-197. doi: 10.1161/CIRCULATIONAHA.116.022010.

[27] Seeburger J, Rinaldi M, Nielsen SL et al. Off-pump transapical implantation of artificial neochordae to correct mitral regurgitation: the TACT trial (Transapical Artificial Chordae Tendinae)proof of concept. J Am Coll Cardiol 2014; 63: 914-9. doi: 10.1016/j.jacc.2013.07.090.

[28] Ramlawi B, Gammie JS. Mitral valve surgery: Current minimally invasive and transcatheter options. Methodist Debakey Cardiovasc J 2016; (1): 20-6. doi: 10.14797/mdcj-12-1-20.

[29] Fiocco A, Nadali M, Speziali G, Colli A. Transcatheter mitral valve chordal repair: Current indications and future perspectives. Front Cardiovasc Med 2019; 6: 128. doi: 10.3389/fcvm.2019.00128

Section 4

New Advances in Minimally Invasive Surgery

Chapter 7

Wearable Technology for Assessment and Surgical Assistance in Minimally Invasive Surgery

Juan A. Sánchez-Margallo, José Castillo Rabazo, Carlos Plaza de Miguel, Peter Gloor, David Durán Rey, Manuel Ramón González-Portillo, Isabel López Agudelo and Francisco M. Sánchez-Margallo

Abstract

Wearable technology is an emerging field that has the potential to revolutionize healthcare. Advances in sensors, augmented reality devices, the internet of things, and artificial intelligence offer clinically relevant and promising functionalities in the field of surgery. Apart from its well-known benefits for the patient, minimally invasive surgery (MIS) is a technically demanding surgical discipline for the surgeon. In this regard, wearable technology has been used in various fields of application in MIS such as the assessment of the surgeon's ergonomic conditions, interaction with the patient or the quality of surgical performance, as well as in providing tools for surgical planning and assistance during surgery. The aim of this chapter is to provide an overview based on the scientific literature and our experience regarding the use of wearable technology in MIS, both in experimental and clinical settings.

Keywords: Sensors, Augmented Reality, Mixed Reality, Internet of Things, Minimally Invasive Surgery

1. Introduction

There is a wide variety of wearable devices, such as smartwatches, wearable mobile sensors, mobile hub medical devices, among others. This technology makes it possible to collect data on the user's health status. A widespread example of the use of this technology is the detection systems of blood glucose levels in diabetic patients [1]. However, wearable technology has also been used in other fields of clinical application, such as minimally invasive surgery (MIS). In this case, this type of technology could make it possible to evaluate the surgeon's ergonomic conditions, the interaction with the patient or the quality of the surgical performance, as well as to provide tools for medical training and surgical assistance.

Apart from the numerous advantages of MIS for the patient, these surgical techniques present several limitations for the surgeon. Some of these challenges include the loss of depth perception due to two-dimensional vision, awkward postures during surgery due to restricted movements, and decreased tactile sensation. All this leads to an increased mental and physical burden on the surgeon during surgery, as well as the possible onset of musculoskeletal disorders. The constant evolution of wearable technology allows for a comprehensive analysis of these parameters in order to improve the surgeon's ergonomics during surgery, and therefore the patient's surgical outcomes [2, 3].

Medical education is a long and demanding process which involves learning complex theoretical and practical aspects. During its early stages, training methods are often based on static and unrealistic learning content. Currently, these methods are being replaced thanks to advances in information and communication technologies. In this regard, new technologies, such as virtual reality (VR), augmented reality (AR), and mixed reality (MR), present the potential to provide medical students with interactive and realistic training contents using head mounted displays (HMD) [4].

During surgical training, the assessment of the technical surgical skills to be acquired by novice surgeons has traditionally been performed by expert surgeons, being a subjective assessment that may be biased. Recent advances in the Internet of Things (IoT), the ability to embed sensors in objects and environments to collect large amounts of data, and advances in machine learning allow for a more objective and automated assessment of MIS skills [5].

On the other hand, advances in preoperative imaging systems have made it a fundamental element in surgical planning [6, 7]. In particular, when facing complex surgeries, surgical planning provides valuable information to predict and reduce any potential risks during surgery, thus improving its safety levels. The application of wearable technology (mainly HMD) in this area provides the surgical team with access to this information in situ and without compromising the asepsis of the surgical procedure [8]. The use of three-dimensional (3D) representations of this data in immersive environments provides new ways to explore the patient information and further enhance the tools available to medical professionals in several areas, such as medical training, surgical planning and intraoperative guidance.

In this chapter we will review some of the aforementioned technologies and medical applications, both described in the scientific literature and those developed by our research group.

2. Evaluation of surgeon's ergonomics

2.1 Physiological parameters

Physiological sensing remains one of the most challenging topics in minimally invasive biomedical signal acquisition today. The clinical gold standard protocols needed to measure biochemical and physiological parameters often require invasive and time-consuming techniques, thus lacking the real-time and comfort factor requirements present in wearable technology.

To date, the most commonly used physiological parameters in the context of wearable technology are still heart rate variability (HRV) [9], as a function of heart rate, and galvanic skin response [10]. Other alternatives are biomarker analysis measured from eccrine sweat [11] and saliva [12], as well as the well-known electroencephalogram (EEG) [13] and surface electromyography (sEMG) [14] techniques.

Smartwatches in particular present a suitable solution as they offer the possibility of acquiring heart rate and motion data simultaneously from the user. Although heart rate sensors included in smartwatches are not adequate for medical

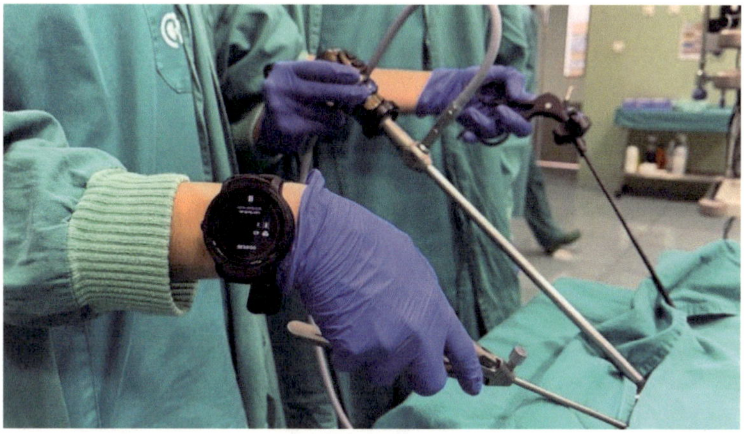

Figure 1.
Smartwatch being used during laparoscopy to acquire surgeon's hand motion and HR.

use or diagnosis, they offer a quick and affordable approach to measure parameters like HRV.

In MIS field, we have made use of smartwatches (**Figure 1**) to monitor hand motion and HRV data of surgeons during the performance of laparoscopic training tasks. Apart from evaluating the surgeon's physiological parameters and performance, we sought to build a machine learning model that could predict stressful situations and quality of surgical performance during laparoscopic practice [2, 15]. Although more data is required in order to build a reliable model, smartwatches are proving to be a promising alternative to more invasive and expensive solutions that are often used in these types of studies.

2.1.1 Muscular activity

The level of effort involved in performing work tasks in a given job is a risk factor for musculoskeletal pathologies. In this sense, different instrumental techniques and wearable systems have been used to evaluate this factor, such as sEMG. Surface electromyography makes it possible to characterize the intensity of muscular intervention of a particular muscle and to identify the onset of muscle fatigue [3]. In the surgical setting, in a study by Wong et al. [16] it was observed that 83% of surgeons showed musculoskeletal symptoms during microlaryngeal surgery, especially in the neck and upper back. However, the assessment of fatigue in microsurgical techniques is especially difficult due to the minimal range of body movement and the low amount of muscle activation required for the performance of the surgical tasks, making them challenging to analyze.

We have studied the effect of experimental microsurgery training on surgeon ergonomics. For this purpose, a total of ten surgeons of different levels of surgical experience were evaluated during the performance of eleven anastomoses in a simulator. A wireless sEMG system (Delsys Trigno; Natick, MA, USA) was used to evaluate the muscle activation of the analyzed muscles (paravertebral, upper trapezius, lower lumbar, and supinator longus muscles) (**Figure 2**). All surgeons showed improvement in their surgical performance. The results revealed that novice surgeons showed, on average, a higher level of muscle activation than intermediate and expert surgeons. In addition, novice surgeons showed greater activation in the muscles on their dominant side, whereas expert surgeons had similar levels of activation on both sides.

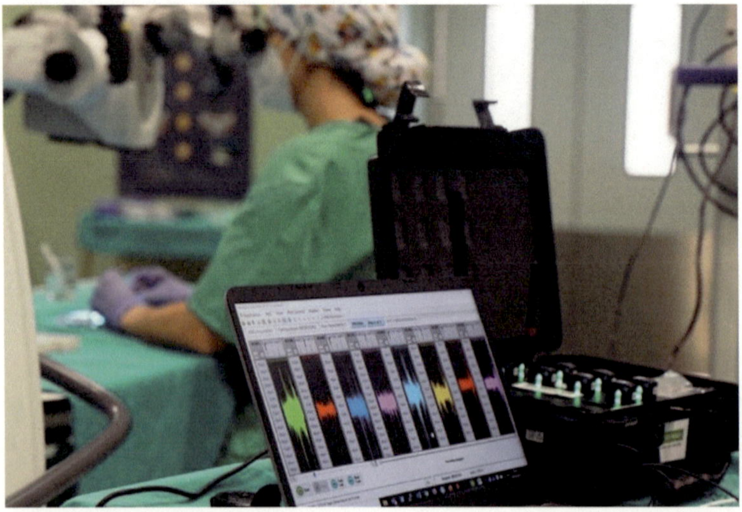

Figure 2.
Use of the Delsys Trigno™ EMG wireless system as a tool for recording sEMG and motion data to assess the surgeon's posture and workload in microsurgery.

2.2 Kinematic parameters

The adoption of forced postures for prolonged periods of time is one of the well-known limitations of laparoscopic surgery. This is why the analysis and evaluation of the working conditions in the operating room (OR) is essential to improve the its ergonomics during MIS. To perform these ergonomic studies, which have traditionally used techniques including photogrammetry and cumbersome EMG systems, techniques based on wearable technologies such as body tracking systems, data gloves, electrogoniometers, smart devices or pressure sensors are now being used [3, 17]. The ultimate goal is to provide practical objective and reliable ergonomic criteria during surgical activity.

Kinematic parameters are associated with the motion of body parts. The technology related to kinematics has been widely studied and implemented in multiple fields as diverse as aeronautics, navigation, video games, or health, among others. Several approaches can be found depending on the needs of the clinical application. The most popular include the use of acceleration sensors, followed by optical tracking solutions. These solutions range from a simple and affordable smartwatch that can measure a subject's hand accelerations from accelerometer sensors [2], to more complex and expensive systems such as the Xsens™ (Xsens Technologies B.V.) that uses inertial sensors [17].

2.2.1 Full body posture

The application of wearable technology for the analysis of full body posture is carried out using markers or sensors placed on the subject's body to quantify the movements of the different body segments. In the case of optical tracking techniques, use is made of a set of retroreflective markers identified by a system of cameras and infrared light [17]. The main limitation of these solutions is the occlusions they may have in the working environment, which is worsened in crowded settings such as an OR.

In recent years, the introduction of inertial sensors has facilitated the application of kinematic analysis techniques in more complex environments as the OR.

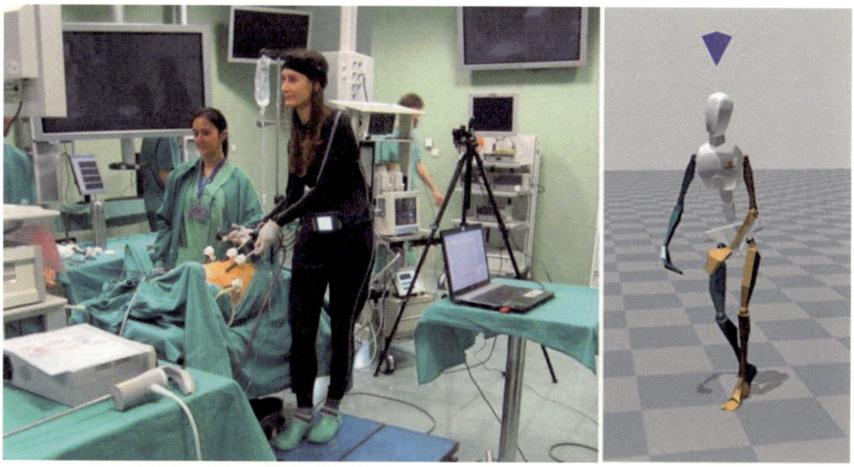

Figure 3.
Motion tracking system based on inertial sensors placed on the surgeon's body (left). A biomechanical model of the subject is created in real time (right). (Source: [17]).

These inertial measurement systems are not affected by visual occlusions, making them suitable for clinical settings (**Figure 3**). This is a more efficient instrumental technique for postural characterization in MIS than conventional techniques such as 3D photogrammetry [3]. In this sense, a study was carried out in which the body posture of 8 laparoscopic surgeons (4 novices and 4 experts) was analyzed by means of the Xsens™ system during the performance of laparoscopic suturing tasks. The kinematic results showed a high variability of the surgeons' body posture, with a coefficient of variation greater than 70% in all the joints, especially in flexion-extension of the wrist and its radial and ulnar deviation [3].

2.2.2 Hand posture

Surgical tasks and instruments directly affect the position of the surgeon's wrist and hand. Data gloves allow comprehensive analysis of the subject's hand movements (**Figure 4A**). Typically, such systems employ electromechanical technology or conductive sensors.

In the clinical setting, the CyberGlove™ system (CyberGlove Systems, San José, CA, USA) has been used to analyze the surgeon's hand movements while using different surgical instruments during laparoscopic practice [18]. The data were analyzed according to an adaptation of the Rapid Upper Limb Assessment (RULA) ergonomic evaluation method. In this study, the hand posture of experienced surgeons in laparoscopic surgery was analyzed during the handling of various handle designs for laparoscopic instruments: axial, axial with rings, and pistol. For all handle designs analyzed, most of the surgeons showed unfavorable flexion-extension angles, with the pistol handle being the most ergonomically suitable design. In another study, instruments for laparoendoscopic single-site surgery (LESS) were found to be ergonomically more suitable than conventional laparoscopic instruments [19].

Wrist flexion-extension and radioulnar deviation during surgical practice can also be recorded using electrogoniometers (**Figure 4B**). These are devices whose measurement signals (usually electrical voltages) are directly related to flexion-extension or rotation between body segments. They must be precalibrated to relate the measured voltage to the angles described by the analyzed joint. As with data gloves, the information provided by electrogoniometers would allow us to

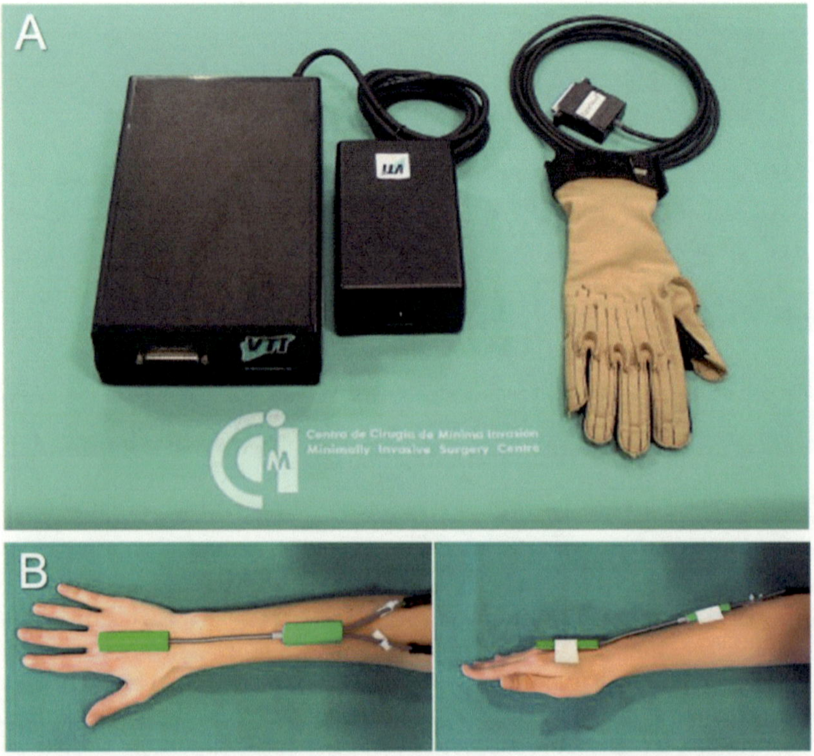

Figure 4.
Use of the CyberGlove™ device (A) and an electrogoniometer (B) for recording the surgeon's hand posture during laparoscopic practice. (Source: [17]).

measure the degree of risk of the surgeon's posture. However, in both cases these devices are difficult to integrate into the surgical environment, and are relegated mainly to experimental studies. This technology has been used to objectively study the surgeon's wrist posture in the use of new handle designs for laparoscopic instruments [20].

2.2.3 Human-instrument interaction

Another relevant risk factor in the surgical context is the localized contact pressure during the use of laparoscopic instruments. Excessive pressure, repeatedly or for long periods of time, can result in nerve damage to the surgeon's fingers. In order to analyze this factor during laparoscopic practice and thus potentially improve the ergonomic conditions of the surgeon and the design of the surgical instruments, wearable systems such as the FingerTPS™ (Pressure Profile Systems, Inc., Hawthorne, CA, USA) can be used. This system makes it possible to measure and map the contact pressures exerted on or by the fingers and the palm of the hand when using the laparoscopic tools (**Figure 5**). This technology makes it possible to assess whether pressure levels are detrimental to the surgeon and to draw conclusions about the most appropriate design for the laparoscopic instruments.

In a study, we evaluated the pressure exerted by the surgeon's distal phalanges of the thumb and the index, middle and ring fingers, as well as the palm of the hand during the use of new handle designs for laparoscopic instruments and with different sizes [20]. The participating surgeons performed three laparoscopic basic tasks to analyze the influence of handle size. The results showed that there was a significant increase in palmar pressure with the incorrectly sized instrument handle.

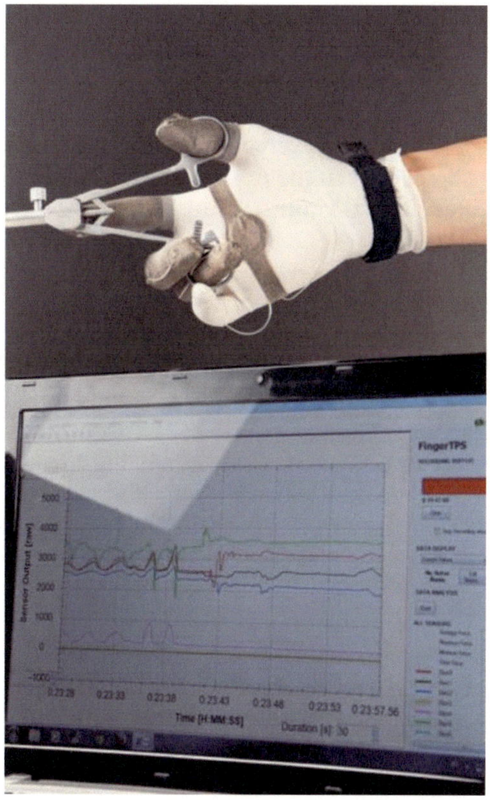

Figure 5.
Use of the FingerTPS™ system during the handling of laparoscopic instruments with a ring handle. (Source: [3]).

On the other hand, in another study we compared the grip pressure in the use of a robotic laparoscopic instrument (Dex Device™; Dex Surgical, Verrières-le-Buisson, France) with respect to conventional laparoscopic tools during urethrovesical anastomosis in experimental model [3]. The results showed that the pressure exerted by the thumb was significantly higher during the use of the robotic instrument. This was due to the interaction with the controls installed on the instrument handle. Additionally, the results showed that the force exerted by the distal phalanx of the index finger was significantly higher with the conventional handle. The palm of the hand was the area that received the greatest pressure while using both instruments.

3. Telementoring and surgical assistance

3.1 Telementoring

Telementoring, defined as mentoring by means of telecommunications and computer networks, allows an experienced physician to directly provide information and share knowledge at a distance with a less experienced practitioner. This is a safe modality for delivering intraoperative surgical education and provides some equivalence to on-site mentoring with regard to clinical and educational outcomes [21].

Meijer et al. demonstrated the feasibility of using wearable technology in combination with the TedCube device (TedCas Medical Systems; Pamplona, Spain) for hands-free interaction with the computer during the course of surgery and for telementoring purposes. The combination of wearable sensors, an integrating device and internet-based remote desktop sharing software proved a feasible set-up for telementoring in situations when asepsis for both the mentor and the mentee is necessary, and distance needs to be overcome. A successful connection without any downtime was established between the Academic Medical Center in Amsterdam, The Netherlands, and Jesús Usón Minimally Invasive Surgery Centre (JUMISC) in Cáceres, Spain [22].

3.2 Surgical assistance

In MIS, preoperative imaging studies are fundamental to facilitate diagnosis and surgical planning. These personalized patient studies allow analysis of anatomical details prior to surgery, improving the course of the procedure. However, surgical environments require very strict aseptic conditions. This makes it difficult to use traditional interaction devices such as keyboard and mouse to consult preoperative patient information during surgery. In addition, some equipment requires the surgeon to leave the OR to access preoperative images, which hinders the surgical process.

The use of wearable systems could offer suitable solutions to these limitations and help maintain surgeon asepsis while interacting with the patient's preoperative data during surgery. One possible device is the MYO armband (Thalmic Labs Inc., Kitchener, ON, Canada), which is worn on the arm (placed just below the elbow). The MYO is equipped with 8 EMG sensors that allow it to recognize the user's hand gestures and arm movements. In a study during the development of several laparoscopic procedures, we demonstrated the feasibility of using a gestural control system by means of the MYO device in conjunction with voice commands to interact with the patient's preoperative imaging studies while maintaining aseptic conditions [23].

4. Head-mounted displays

Head-mounted displays (HMD) are, of all the devices that allow viewing digital content, the ones that achieve greater user immersion in digital content. Technologies such as stereoscopy (projecting a different image of the same environment in each eye, thus achieving a sense of depth) allow user immersion in a virtual environment. The possibility of using hand gestures, voice commands or eye-tracking devices that allow interaction with the environment represents a paradigm shift since, without these elements, HMDs would be passive devices, being able only to display content but not to interact with it.

These wearable devices allow the visualization of content through different types of technologies [24]. At one extreme is Virtual Reality (VR) where all the content displayed is completely digital and the real environment is ignored. At the other extreme is Augmented Reality (AR), in which the environment is visualized and layers of digital information are added based on what is seen. Mixed Reality (MR) is in the middle ground, as it displays computer-generated content that is aware of the environment, allowing users to interact with the content but taking into account the environment around them. VR can be a useful tool for various simulators or educational applications, although it has limitations in terms of assistance during surgical applications (**Figure 6**).

Until 2016, Google Glasses (Google Inc.; Mountain View, California, USA) [25] was the most widely used HMD for viewing digital content. However, several

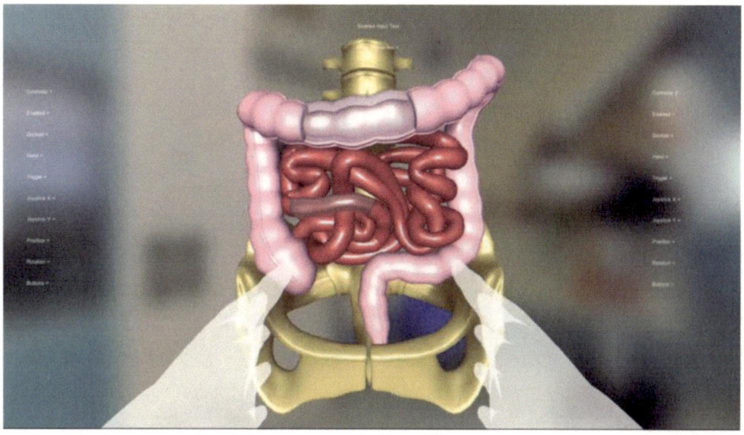

Figure 6.
VR application oriented to anatomical education.

publications have mentioned the limitations of this device for its application in the medical field. Some of them are its restricted functionalities, low computational capacity, poor display resolution, information projected on a single eye (which negates stereoscopy), and usability limitations due to its incompatibility with the use of glasses or privacy aspects [26]. Over time, MR devices have become a standard, as they allow the inclusion of holographic images or 3D objects, which are displayed in the user's field of view and integrated with the real environment, improving the immersive experience during work.

4.1 Surgical training

In the educational field, most VR applications dedicated to surgeon training have a fully immersive nature, due to the inherent characteristics of this type of technology. Simulation using devices such as Oculus Rift (Oculus VR; Menlo Park, CA, USA) offers complete immersion and VR controls mimic the surgeon's surgical tools [27]. Other applications are able to offer a much more detailed visualization of the human anatomy using HMD devices such as HTC Vive (HTC Corporation; Xindian, Taiwan) [28]. In most cases, this methodology offers possibilities for training outside the OR, collecting surgical performance metrics from the user as if it were a serious game [29]. These solutions allow procedures to be repeated without any restriction, reducing training costs [30], and obtaining also progression feedback for each user, thus enabling the improvement of less developed surgical skills.

In the case of Google Glass, these have been used mainly as a means of sharing with students the surgeon's view during his/her performance, along with real-time comments, which allows the generation of comprehensive content for learning [31]. Finally, it is worth mentioning the use of this device together with an ultrasound probe for the visualization of the 3D ultrasound images generated, facilitating the learning of human anatomy [32].

Regarding AR/MR devices, most training applications are based on the visualization of anatomical elements [33]. As the main potential of these technologies lies in knowing the environment and coupling spatially augmented information to it, numerous applications opt for using visual markers and superimposing digital content on them [34]. On the other hand, it is worth highlighting the wide possibilities offered by these devices in telemedicine and remote medical training [35]. This technology offers a significant improvement in 3D perception compared to two-dimensional illustrations or more traditional training content (**Figure 7A**).

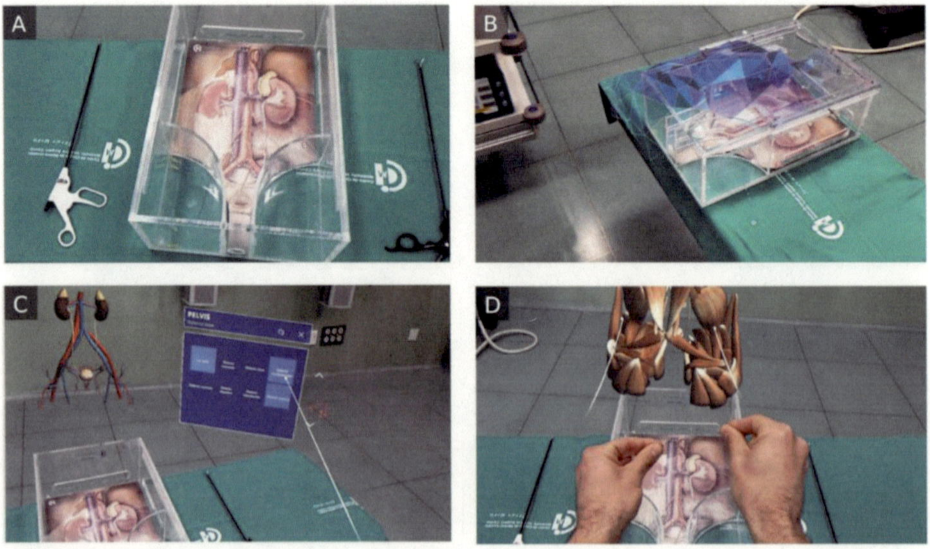

Figure 7.
MR application for anatomical training: (A) traditional simulator with medical illustrations; (B) spatial detection of the simulator using the HoloLens depth camera; (C) selection of the anatomical element to be displayed; (D) example of gestural interaction with the 3D hologram.

MR devices, such as HoloLens (Microsoft; Redmond, Washington, USA), make it possible to scan the working environment (**Figure 7B**) and provide 3D anatomical models, as well as organize them into different systems (nervous, muscle, bone, or vascular) (**Figure 7C**). The user can interact (move, rotate or scale) with the holograms by means of gestures or voice commands (**Figure 7D**). These applications have been tested in various contexts by expert surgeons at the JUMISC, concluding that the visualization of 3D anatomical models using this technology is useful and facilitates the transfer of knowledge to real clinical practice [36].

4.2 Surgical assistance

In relation to surgical assistance, Google Glass emerged as a means of broadcasting the surgeon's vision for telementoring applications and requesting expert opinion outside the OR [37]. On the other hand, this device has also been used to provide the endoscopic image in place of traditional laparoscopic monitors. Another surgical assistance application is the display of checklists to proceed in a more orderly and safe way with the surgical procedure [38]. Various sensors of this device (camera, microphone) have also been exploited in combination with other devices such as Fitbit™ (Fitbit, San Francisco, California, USA) to collect data and facilitate surgical evaluation and performance [39]. Of note is the feasibility, safety and usability study by Borgmann et al. in which preoperative studies were shown during ten types of urological surgery procedures [40].

Since 2016, the use of Microsoft's HoloLens glasses has been gaining presence in the field of AR applied to surgery to the detriment of Google Glass. This device marked a milestone in AR HMD devices, even defining a new term (mixed reality -MR-) since, due to the built-in depth cameras, the device is aware of both the surrounding spatial environment (**Figure 8A** and **D**) and the gestures that the user performs with the hands even when holding the surgical tools (**Figure 8B** and **C**), thus resulting in a more complete integration of the information displayed on the glasses with the OR. The nature of this device makes it an exceptional choice for use

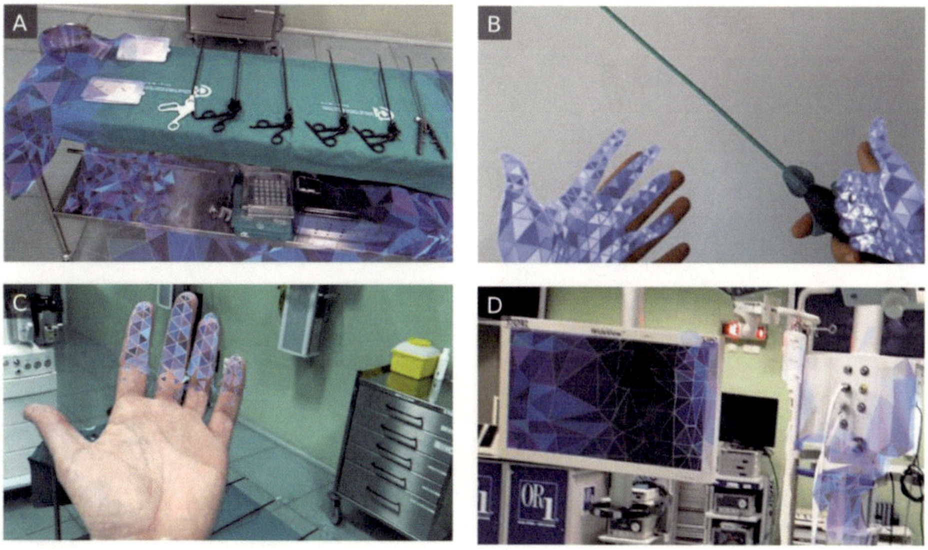

Figure 8.
MR application for surgical assistance: spatial detection of the surgical environment (A and D); detection of the surgeon's hand gestures (B and C).

in surgical assisting applications. Recently, applications have been presented on the use of this type of device in MIS, in kidney and prostate surgical procedures [41], lung, and uterus [42], among others.

The Remote Assist application (Microsoft) for HoloLens has recently been presented, which could facilitate medical training and telementoring tasks. This application is capable of video calls sharing the surgeon's point of view, allowing both communicating surgical knowledge with trainees and consulting with clinical experts in real time. The application accesses the depth camera to spatially locate 3D elements in the OR environment, allowing to point out elements such as surgical material or equipment or to explain the operation of the equipment in an intuitive way (**Figure 9**). In addition, the user using the device is be able to see the expert/apprentice in the form of a hologram (**Figure 9D**). Due to the recent need for distance learning/mentoring solutions, these tools are emerging as useful alternatives.

MR technology can also be used for surgical planning. It could facilitate visualization and analysis of the patient's preoperative imaging studies for a better and safer approach to surgery. MR devices, in combination with new emerging medical imaging techniques, have been successfully applied as a planning tool in different surgical disciplines such as urology [43], thoracic surgery [44], neurosurgery, colorectal surgery, and bariatric surgery [45], among others.

Surgeons can interact with the 3D models generated from preoperative studies of the patient for a better understanding of the anatomy to be operated on (**Figure 10B**). Recent studies have managed to visualize in real time the preoperative studies stored in DICOM format, allowing a more complete and interactive view in the form of a hologram. These applications make it possible to visualize the preoperative imaging study based on the density of each point, as well as to perform filters on the point cloud (**Figure 10A**, **C** and **D**). We have used this surgical planning application during a laparoscopic renal tumorectomy in experimental model [46] and during a laparoscopic lobectomy at the University Hospital of Cáceres (Spain) [47]. Surgeons highlighted the usefulness of the application for planning laparoscopic procedures, although they also reported some ergonomic limitation of the MR device.

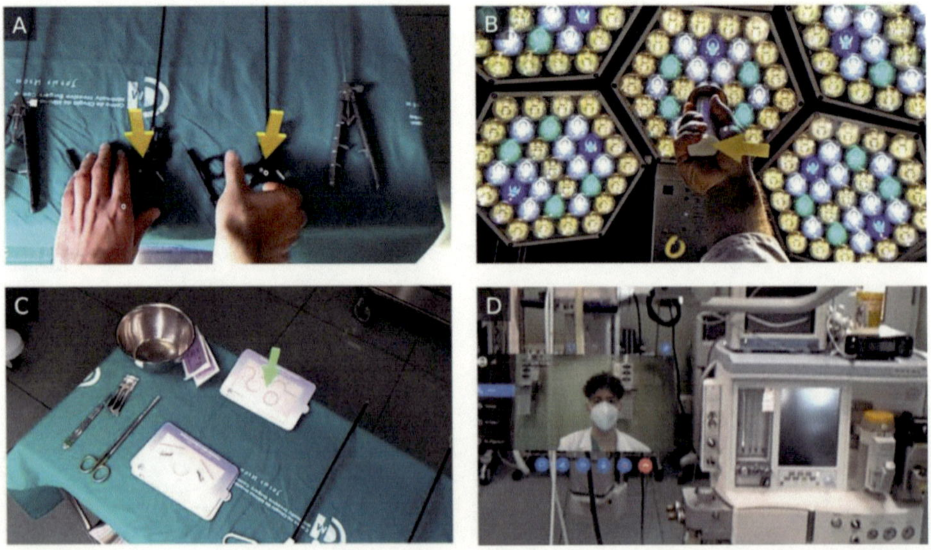

Figure 9.
Use of the Remote Assist (Microsoft) application: spatial markers (A–C); video call sharing the surgeon's point of view (D).

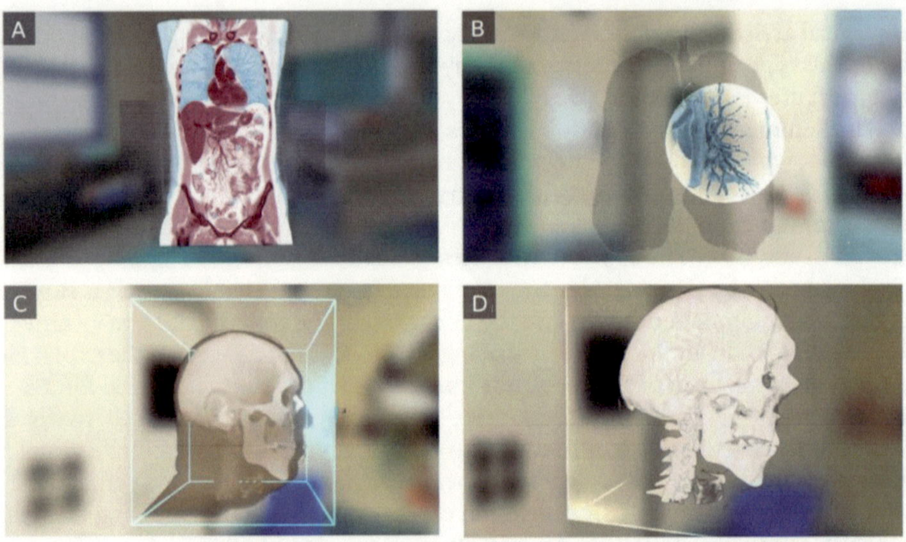

Figure 10.
MR application used to visualize preoperative studies: Visualization of the volumetric point cloud (A, C, D); visualization of the 3D model (B).

Another application of this technology for surgical assistance is its use as an additional monitor during surgery. Ten surgeons evaluated this function during the performance of a simple laparoscopic training task (object transfer task) (**Figure 11A**, **C** and **D**). For this purpose, the participants used the HoloLens v2 glasses as a holographic monitor, instead of a conventional laparoscopic monitor. Most surgeons concluded that they could perform more complex tasks using the holographic monitor. The application achieved positive results in terms of latency, image quality and user experience. The surgeons showed a slight learning curve when it came to spatially positioning the monitor (**Figure 11B**), mainly due to the fact that in most cases it was their first experience with this type of device.

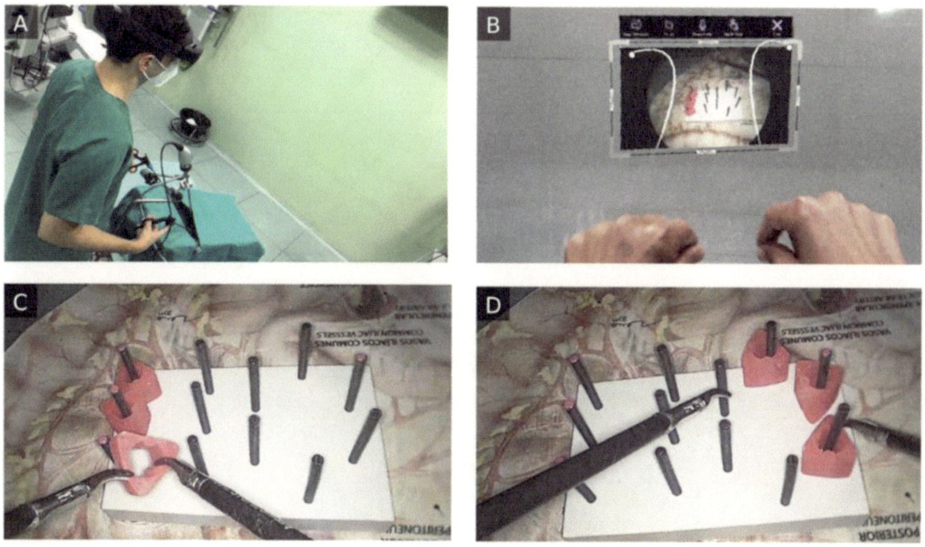

Figure 11.
Use of MR application as a holographic monitor during laparoscopic practice: setting of the study (A); positioning and scaling of the holographic monitor (B); start and end of the transfer task (C and D).

5. Conclusions

The constant evolution of wearable technology has boosted its application in the surgical field, especially in minimally invasive surgery. This technology allows an exhaustive analysis of the surgeon's physiological and ergonomic conditions during the surgical practice, improving the surgeon health and surgical equipment design, and therefore surgical outcomes for the patient. On the other hand, this technology has led to a paradigm shift in medical training, taking the student to the same operating room in which an intervention is being performed or offering holographic and interactive 3D anatomical models close to reality. In addition, head-mounted displays offer surgeons advanced tools for surgical planning, providing access to the patient's preoperative information in the operating room, while maintaining aseptic conditions. Undoubtedly, developments in sensors, data analysis techniques, artificial intelligence and mixed reality will continue to offer new and innovative solutions to clinical needs.

Acknowledgements

This study has been partially funded by the MISTI Global Seed Funds, "la Caixa" Foundation, Junta de Extremadura (Spain), European Social Fund, European Regional Development Fund (ERDF) "A way to make Europe", and the Spanish Ministry of Science, Innovation and Universities through ERDF funds of the Intelligent Growth Operational Program (LCF/PR/MIT18/11830006, TA18023, PD18077, GR18199, CPI-2019-2033-1-TRE –14).

Conflict of interest

The authors declare no conflict of interest.

Author details

Juan A. Sánchez-Margallo[1*], José Castillo Rabazo[1], Carlos Plaza de Miguel[1], Peter Gloor[2], David Durán Rey[1], Manuel Ramón González-Portillo[1], Isabel López Agudelo[1] and Francisco M. Sánchez-Margallo[1]

1 Jesús Usón Minimally Invasive Surgery Centre, Cáceres, Spain

2 MIT Centre for Collective Intelligence, MA, USA

*Address all correspondence to: jasanchez@ccmijesususon.com

References

[1] Dinh-Le C, Chuang R, Chokshi S, Mann D. Wearable Health Technology and Electronic Health Record Integration: Scoping Revie7w and Future Directions. JMIR Mhealth Uhealth. 2019;7(9):e12861.

[2] Sánchez-Margallo JA, Gloor PA, Campos JL, Sánchez-Margallo FM. Measuring Workload and Performance of Surgeons Using Body Sensors of Smartwatches. In: Digital Transformation of Collaboration. Springer; 2020. p. 67-74.

[3] Gianikellis K, Skiadopoulos A, Horrillo RG, Rodal M, Sánchez-margallo JA, Sánchez-margallo FM. Advanced Ergonomics in Laparoscopic Surgery. In: Sánchez-Margallo FM, Sánchez-Margallo JA, editors. Recent Advances in Laparoscopic Surgery. IntechOpen; 2019. p. 1-23.

[4] Lahanas V, Loukas C, Smailis N, Georgiou E. A novel augmented reality simulator for skills assessment in minimal invasive surgery. Surg Endosc. 2015 Aug;29(8):2224-2234.

[5] Castillo-Segura P, Fernández-Panadero C, Alario-Hoyos C, Muñoz-Merino PJ, Delgado Kloos C. Objective and automated assessment of surgical technical skills with IoT systems: A systematic literature review. Artif Intell Med. 2021 Feb;112(November 2020):102007.

[6] Sánchez-Margallo FM, Sánchez-Margallo JA. Computer-Assisted Minimally Invasive Surgery: Image-Guided Interventions and Robotic Surgery. In: Xiaojun Chen, editor. Computer-Assisted Surgery. Nova Science Publishers, Inc.; 2015. p. 43-94.

[7] Smith RT, Clarke TJ, Mayer W, Cunningham A, Matthews B, Zucco JE. Mixed Reality Interaction and Presentation Techniques for Medical Visualisations. Adv Exp Med Biol. 2020;1260:123-139.

[8] Sadeghi AH, Bakhuis W, Van Schaagen F, Oei FBS, Bekkers JA, Maat APWM, et al. Immersive 3D virtual reality imaging in planning minimally invasive and complex adult cardiac surgery. Eur Hear J - Digit Heal. 2020;1(1):62-70.

[9] Graham SA, Jeste DV, Lee EE, Wu TC, Tu X, Kim HC, et al. Associations between heart rate variability measured with a wrist-worn sensor and older adults' physical function: observational study. JMIR Mhealth Uhealth. 2019 Oct 23;7(10):e13757.

[10] Yoon S, Sim JK, Cho YH. A Flexible and Wearable Human Stress Monitoring Patch. Sci Rep. 2016 Mar 23;6:23468.

[11] Sonner Z, Wilder E, Heikenfeld J, Kasting G, Beyette F, Swaile D, et al. The microfluidics of the eccrine sweat gland, including biomarker partitioning, transport, and biosensing implications. Biomicrofluidics. 2015 May 15;9(3):031301.

[12] Chiappin S, Antonelli G, Gatti R, De Palo EF. Saliva specimen: a new laboratory tool for diagnostic and basic investigation. Clin Chim Acta. 2007 Aug;383(1-2):30-40.

[13] Zhang X, Li J, Liu Y, Zhang Z, Wang Z, Luo D, et al. Design of a Fatigue Detection System for High-Speed Trains Based on Driver Vigilance Using a Wireless Wearable EEG. Sensors (Basel). 2017 Mar 1;17(3):486.

[14] Biagetti G, Crippa P, Falaschetti L, Orcioni S, Turchetti C. Human activity monitoring system based on wearable sEMG and accelerometer wireless sensor nodes. Biomed Eng Online. 2018 Nov 20;17(Suppl 1):132.

[15] Sánchez-Margallo FM, Gloor P, Durán Rey D, Sánchez-Margallo JA. Uso de dispositivos inteligentes para la predicción de la carga de trabajo durante la práctica laparoscópica. Cir Esp. 2020;98(Espec Congr 1):471

[16] Wong A, Baker N, Smith L, Rosen CA. Prevalence and risk factors for musculoskeletal problems associated with microlaryngeal surgery: a national survey. Laryngoscope. 2014 Aug;124(8):1854-1861.

[17] Sánchez-Margallo FM, Sánchez-Margallo JA. Ergonomics in Laparoscopic Surgery. In: Malik AM, editor. Laparoscopic Surgery. London: InTech; 2017. p. 105-123.

[18] Sánchez-Margallo FM, Sánchez-Margallo JA, Pagador JB, Moyano JL, Moreno J, Usón J. Ergonomic Assessment of Hand Movements in Laparoscopic Surgery Using the CyberGlove. In: Miller K, Nielsen PMF, editors. Computational Biomechanics for Medicine. New York, NY: Springer New York; 2010. p. 121-128.

[19] Pérez-Duarte FJ, Lucas-Hernández M, Matos-Azevedo A, Sánchez-Margallo JA, Díaz-Güemes I, Sánchez-Margallo FM. Objective analysis of surgeons' ergonomy during laparoendoscopic single-site surgery through the use of surface electromyography and a motion capture data glove. Surg Endosc. 2014;28(4):1314-1320.

[20] Sánchez-Margallo JA, González González A, García Moruno L, Gómez-Blanco JC, Pagador JB, Sánchez-Margallo FM. Comparative Study of the Use of Different Sizes of an Ergonomic Instrument Handle for Laparoscopic Surgery. Appl Sci. 2020 Feb 24;10(4):1526.

[21] Erridge S, Yeung DKT, Patel HRH, Purkayastha S. Telementoring of Surgeons: A Systematic Review. Surg Innov. 2019 Feb;26(1):95-111.

[22] Meijer HAW, Sánchez Margallo JA, Sánchez Margallo FM, Goslings JC, Schijven MP. Wearable technology in an international telementoring setting during surgery: a feasibility study. BMJ Innov. 2017;3(4):189-195.

[23] Sánchez-Margallo FM, Sánchez-Margallo JA, Moyano-Cuevas JL, Pérez EM, Maestre J. Use of natural user interfaces for image navigation during laparoscopic surgery: initial experience. Minim Invasive Ther Allied Technol. 2017 Sep 3;26(5):253-261.

[24] Kamarudin B, Fadzil M, Nabil Z. Augmented Reality, Virtual Reality and Mixed Reality in Medical Education: A Comparative Web of Science Scoping Review. Preprints. 2019; 2019040323.

[25] Wei NJ, Dougherty B, Myers A, Badawy SM. Using Google Glass in Surgical Settings: Systematic Review. JMIR Mhealth Uhealth. 2018 Mar 6;6(3):e54.

[26] Kolodzey L, Grantcharov P, Rivas H,Schijven M, Grantcharov T. Wearable technology in the operating room: A systematic review. BMJ Innov. 2017;3:55-63.

[27] Mathur A. Low cost virtual reality for medical training. 2015 IEEE Virtual Reality (VR). 2015;345-346.

[28] Egger J, Gall M, Wallner J, Boechat P, Hann A, Li X, et al. HTC Vive MeVisLab integration via OpenVR for medical applications. PLoS One. 2017 Mar 21;12(3):e0173972.

[29] Grantcharov TP, Kristiansen VB, Bendix J, Bardram L, Rosenberg J, Funch-Jensen P. Randomized clinical trial of virtual reality simulation for laparoscopic skills training. Br J Surg. 2004 Feb;91(2):146-150.

[30] de Visser H, Watson MO, Salvado O, Passenger JD. Progress in virtual reality simulators for surgical training and certification. Med J Aust. 2011 Feb 21;194(4):S38-S40.

[31] Rahimy E, Garg SJ. Google Glass for recording scleral buckling surgery. JAMA Ophthalmol. 2015; 133:710-711.

[32] Benninger B. Google Glass, ultrasound and palpation: the anatomy teacher of the future? Clin Anat. 2015 Mar;28(2):152-155.

[33] Moro C, Phelps C, Redmond P, Štromberga Z. HoloLens and mobile augmented reality in medical and health science education: A randomised controlled trial. Br J Educ Technol. 2020; 52:680-694.

[34] Liebmann F, Roner S, von Atzigen M, Scaramuzza D, Sutter R, Snedeker J, et al. Pedicle screw navigation using surface digitization on the Microsoft HoloLens. Int J Comput Assist Radiol Surg. 2019 Jul;14(7):1157-1165.

[35] Wang S, Parsons M, Stone-McLean J, Rogers P, Boyd S, Hoover K, et al. Augmented Reality as a Telemedicine Platform for Remote Procedural Training. Sensors. 2017;17(10):2294.

[36] Sánchez-Margallo FM, Sánchez-Margallo JA, Cristo A, Rodríguez A, Suárez M. Application of Mixed Reality Technology for Surgical Training in Urology. Surg Endosc. 2018;32:S655.

[37] Hamann D, Mortensen WS, Hamann CR, Smith A, Martino B, Dameff C, Tully J, Kim J, Torres A. Experiences in adoption of teledermatology in Mohs micrographic surgery: using smartglasses for intraoperative consultation and defect triage. Surg Innov. 2014 Dec;21(6):653-654.

[38] Mitrasinovic S, Camacho E, Trivedi N, Logan J, Campbell C, Zilinyi R, Lieber B, Bruce E, Taylor B, Martineau D, Dumont EL, Appelboom G, Connolly ES Jr. Clinical and surgical applications of smart glasses. Technol Health Care. 2015;23(4):381-401.

[39] Pugh CM, Golden RN. Medical Training in the Fitbit, Google Glass and Personal Information Era. WMJ. 2015 Aug;114(4):168-169.

[40] Borgmann H, Rodríguez Socarrás M, Salem J, Tsaur I, Gomez Rivas J, Barret E, Tortolero L. Feasibility and safety of augmented reality-assisted urological surgery using smartglass. World J Urol. 2017 Jun;35(6):967-972.

[41] Amparore D, Pecoraro A, Checcucci E, DE Cillis S, Piramide F, Volpi G, et al. 3D imaging technologies in minimally-invasive kidney and prostate cancer surgery: which is the urologists' perception? Minerva Urol Nephrol. 2021 Mar 26.

[42] Al Janabi HF, Aydin A, Palaneer S, Macchione N, Al-Jabir A, Khan MS, Dasgupta P, Ahmed K. Effectiveness of the HoloLens mixed-reality headset in minimally invasive surgery: a simulation-based feasibility study. Surg Endosc. 2020 Mar;34(3):1143-1149.

[43] Li G, Dong J, Wang J, Cao D, Zhang X, Cao Z, Lu G. The clinical application value of mixed-reality-assisted surgical navigation for laparoscopic nephrectomy. Cancer Med. 2020 Aug;9(15):5480-5489.

[44] Perkins SL, Krajancich B, Yang CJ, Hargreaves BA, Daniel BL, Berry MF. A Patient-Specific Mixed-Reality Visualization Tool for Thoracic Surgical Planning. Ann Thorac Surg. 2020 Jul;110(1):290-295.

[45] Cartucho J, Shapira D, Ashrafian H, Giannarou S. Multimodal mixed reality

visualisation for intraoperative surgical guidance. Int J Comput Assist Radiol Surg. 2020 May;15(5):819-826.

[46] Sánchez-Margallo FM, Sánchez-Margallo JA, Suárez M, Cristo A, Rodríguez A, Moyano-Cuevas JL. Tecnologías de control gestual y realidad aumentada para la asistencia en cirugía de mínima invasión Cir Esp. 2018;96(Espec Congr):1.

[47] Sánchez-Margallo JA, Fernández-Anzules RA, Plaza de Miguel C, Sánchez-Margallo FM. Mixed Reality Application for Surgical Planning in Video-Assisted Pulmonary Lobectomy. Br J Surg. 2021;108(Supplement_3).